CLINICAL ROTATION MANUAL FOR THE ACUTE CARE NURSE PRACTITIONER STUDENT

Nichole Miller, AGACNP-BC, MSN, has over 20 years of nursing experience, primarily in critical care. She is currently a nocturnist at the Joseph M. Still Burn Center in Augusta, Georgia, and visiting faculty for the nurse practitioner program at Chamberlain University. She started her career as an LPN in 2001, and she obtained her BSN in 2010 and an MSN with a focus of nursing education in 2013. Her DNP focused on adult-gerontologic acute care. She has authored several articles and presented at both the Southern Regional Burn Symposium and the American Association of Critical Care Nurses National Teaching Institute.

With a contribution by Tish Myers, MSN, APRN, FNP-BC, Burn and Reconstructive Centers of America, Augusta, Georgia

CLINICAL ROTATION MANUAL FOR THE ACUTE CARE NURSE PRACTITIONER STUDENT

Nichole Miller, AGACNP-BC, MSN

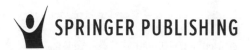

Springer Publishing Company, LLC
11 West 42nd Street, New York, NY 10036
www.springerpub.com
connect.springerpub.com/

Acquisitions Editor: Rachel X. Landes
Compositor: Amnet Systems

ISBN: 978-0-8261-8922-6
ebook ISBN: 978-0-8261-8923-3
DOI: 10.1891/9780826189233

21 22 23 24 / 5 4 3 2 1

The author and the publisher of this work have made every effort to use sources believed to be reliable to provide information that is accurate and compatible with the standards generally accepted at the time of publication. Because medical science is continually advancing, our knowledge base continues to expand. Therefore, as new information becomes available, changes in procedures become necessary. We recommend that the reader always consult current research and specific institutional policies before performing any clinical procedure or delivering any medication. The author and publisher shall not be liable for any special, consequential, or exemplary damages resulting, in whole or in part, from the readers' use of, or reliance on, the information contained in this book. The publisher has no responsibility for the persistence or accuracy of URLs for external or third-party internet websites referred to in this publication and does not guarantee that any content on such websites is, or will remain, accurate or appropriate.

Library of Congress Cataloging-in-Publication Data
Names: Miller, Nichole, author, editor.
Title: Clinical rotation manual for the acute care nurse practitioner student / Nichole Miller.
Description: New York, NY : Springer Publishing Company, LLC, [2022] |
  Includes bibliographical references and index.
Identifiers: LCCN 2021018684 (print) | LCCN 2021018685 (ebook) | ISBN
  9780826189226 (paperback) | ISBN 9780826189233 (ebook)
Subjects: MESI I: Critical Care Nursing—methods | Nurse Practitioners | Outline
Classification: LCC RC86.7 (print) | LCC RC86.7 (ebook) | NLM WY 18.2 | DDC 616.02/8 —dc23
LC record available at https://lccn.loc.gov/2021018684
LC ebook record available at https://lccn.loc.gov/2021018685

Publisher's Note: New and used products purchased from third-party sellers are not guaranteed for quality, authenticity, or access to any included digital components.

Printed in the United States of America.

This book is dedicated to my family.
First to my husband, who has supported me every step of
the way in following my dreams.
To my daughters, who have watched me type while at practice,
dance, and even on vacation.
Thank you for always understanding.
To my parents, thank you for always telling me that anything is possible.
It has kept me going even when I have wanted to give up.
To all the mentors that have helped me grow along the way,
thank you for helping me become the nurse and provider that I am today.

CONTENTS

FOREWORD

This timely book was inspired because of the need for a clinical book that addresses the needs of acute care nurse practitioners. This new book, *Clinical Rotation Manual for the Acute Care Nurse Practitioner*, builds on the work of acute care nurse practitioners over the past 20 years. Chapters cover complex care problems in the acute care setting with the most current evidence-based information. Using an interprofessional approach, this book focuses on clinical decision-making and collaboration.

This manual is divided into chapters by system, beginning with the cardiovascular system and concluding with infectious diseases. Each chapter section is divided into common disease states. The easy-to-read-and-follow book includes clinical tips and tricks, normal lab values, causes, assessment findings, treatment and management methods, and critical-level treatment.

Dr. Miller has included billing, assessments, and documentation in the final section. Templates for documentation and billing are included. Documentation includes a template for history and physicals, tips, and tricks in documentation.

Critically important clinical information on practice is provided. The information provided in this book will provide the foundation needed for new graduates as well as seasoned acute care nurse practitioners information to practice at the highest level of nurse practitioner practice. Dr. Miller has taken great care to write this book in an easy-to-read-and-follow format to meet the needs of acutely ill patients while providing high-quality cost-effective care. This book will act as a resource for the acute care nurse practitioner at a variety of stages, from student to novice to expert.

Mary Ellen Roberts, DNP, APN-C, NP-C, FNAP, FAANP, FAAN
Director—DNP and Acute Care Nurse Practitioner Programs
Seton Hall University
Nutley, New Jersey

PREFACE

Welcome to the *Clinical Rotation Manual for the Acute Care Nurse Practitioner Student.* This book is designed to prepare the acute care nurse practitioner student for those complicated and complex clinical situations you may not have yet explored fully in the didactic part of your program. When I was an acute care nurse practitioner student myself, I recognized that there were no resources specifically designed for the acute care nurse practitioner. As I began my practice and began to precept, I noticed that no new resources had been developed. And after several years of precepting nurse practitioner students, I received a lot of feedback that certain disease processes had not yet been covered in their course work, often leading to frustration and difficulty working through complex differential diagnoses during clinical rotations.

This book has been developed as a bridge to fill those gaps in knowledge and help build confidence in the clinical setting. While no resource will replace those hours of course work, this book will help guide you through some complex clinical situations. This book is organized first by body systems then by disease processes. Each disease process is then broken down into causes, assessment findings, diagnostic testing, and treatment and management sections. This hopefully will allow you to correlate assessment findings, order appropriate diagnostic testing, and identify appropriate management and treatments.

Another key feature of this book is the Clinical Tips and Tricks boxes. These are clinical tips that may help as quick tips or bits of information on certain disease processes. These are important facts and knowledge bits that are used frequently in practice. Areas that are commonly found in practice are often found on tests as well, so it is helpful to know this material.

While this book is meant to be a clinical manual, it can also be a great companion to classroom learning. It takes each complex concept and breaks it down into its very basic parts. As you grow in your knowledge and your practice as a nurse practitioner, you build on your knowledge. This book can be a great building block for those who may benefit from that learning style. I hope you find this book useful and enjoy its contents.

Nichole Miller

ABBREVIATIONS

ACTH	adrenocorticotropic hormone
ADH	antidiuretic hormone
ALT	alanine transaminase
ANA	antinuclear antibody
ARDS	adult respiratory distress syndrome
AST	aspartate transaminase
BNP	brain natriuretic peptide
BP	blood pressure
CABG	coronary artery bypass graft
CAUTI	catheter-associated urinary tract infection
CC	chief complaint
CI	cardiac index
CLABSI	central line blood stream infection
CMV	cytomegalovirus
CO	cardiac output
CRE	carbapenem-resistant enterobacteriaceae
CRP	C-reactive protein
CVP	central venous pressure
DKA	diabetic ketoacidosis
DRESS	drug reaction with eosinophilia and systemic symptoms
EBL	estimated blood loss
EBV	Epstein–Barr virus
EF	ejection fraction
ERCP	endoscopic retrograde cholangio-pancreatography
ESR	eosinophil sedimentary rate
FENa	fraction of excreted sodium
FFP	fresh frozen plasma
FWD	free water deficit
HEENT	head, eyes, ears, nose, and throat
HHS	hyperglycemic hyperosmolar state
HPI	history of present illness
HSV	herpes simplex virus
ICD	intracardiac defibrillators
LDH	lactate dehydrogenase
MAC	monitored anesthesia care
MAP	mean arterial pressure
MI	myocardial infarction

MRSA	methicillin-resistant *Staphylococcus aureus*
MV	minute ventilation
NSTEMI	non-ST elevation myocardial infarction
PCI	percutaneous coronary intervention
PRBC	packed red blood cells
PT	prothrombin time
PTH	parathyroid hormone
ROS	review of systems
SIADH	syndrome of inappropriate diuretic hormone
STEMI	ST elevation myocardial infarction
SVR	systemic vascular resistance
TBW	total body water
TIPSS	transjugular intrahepatic portosystemic shunt
TRALI	transfusion-related acute lung injury
TSH	thyroid stimulating hormone
URI	urinary tract infection
VAP	ventilator-associated pneumonia
VRE	vancomycin-resistant enterococcus
WBC	white blood cells

SECTION I

CARDIOVASCULAR DISEASE AND DISORDERS

ACUTE CORONARY SYNDROME AND MYOCARDIAL INFARCTION

Causes

> ### CLINICAL TIPS AND TRICKS
>
> - Acute coronary syndrome
>   - Diagnosis made when myocardial ischemia is suspected but not yet confirmed
> - Myocardial infarction (MI)
>   - Acute atherosclerotic plaque disruption or abruption
>   - Oxygen supply–demand mismatch
> - Unstable angina
>   - Ischemic symptoms without elevation in biomarkers

- Acute atherosclerotic plaque disruption or abruption
- Oxygen supply–demand mismatch
- Risk factors
  - Family history of sudden cardiac death
  - Coronary artery disease
  - Hyperlipidemia
  - Diabetes
  - Cocaine abuse/use
- ST elevation myocardial infarction (STEMI)
- Non–ST elevation myocardial infarction (NSTEMI)

> ### CLINICAL TIPS AND TRICKS
>
> #### MYOCARDIAL INFARCTION TYPES
>
> **Type I**
>
> - Coronary artery atherothrombosis rupture or disturbance
>
> **Type II**
>
> - Infarction due to supply–demand mismatch
>
> **Type III**
>
> - Sudden death without biomarkers being obtained

(continued)

Type IV

■ Infarction due to previous percutaneous intervention (PCI)

Type V

■ Infarction due to coronary artery bypass graft (CABG) intervention

Assessment Findings

CLINICAL TIPS AND TRICKS

CHEST PAIN: DIFFERENTIAL DIAGNOSES TO CONSIDER

Cardiac

■ Aortic dissection
■ Myocarditis
■ Pericarditis
■ Takotsubo cardiomyopathy

Musculoskeletal

■ Costochondritis
■ Rib fractures
■ Muscle strain

Pulmonary

■ Pneumonia
■ Pleuritis
■ Pulmonary embolism

Psychiatric

■ Anxiety
■ Delusions

Gastrointestinal

■ Cholecystitis
■ Colic
■ Esophagitis
■ Reflux
■ Ulcer

■ Chest pain
  ● Substernal
  ● Epigastric
  ● Often described as crushing
  ● May radiate to the neck or jaw

- Back pain
- Arm pain
- Abdominal pain
- Nausea
- Tachycardia
- Bradycardia
- Arrhythmias
  - Ventricular tachycardia
  - Ventricular fibrillation
- Diaphoresis
- Sudden cardiac death
- Reports of decreased activity tolerance

Diagnostics

CLINICAL TIPS AND TRICKS

EKG CHANGES IN ACUTE MYOCARDIAL INFARCTION

Inferior wall
II, III, aVF

Lateral wall
I, aVL

Anterolateral wall
V5, V6

Anteroapical wall
V3, V4

Anteroseptal wall
V1, V2

EKG
- ST elevations
  - >2-mm elevation in leads V2 and V3
  - >1-mm elevation in leads I, II, III, aVR, aVL, aVF, and V3 to V6
  - Must be in contiguous leads to be significant
- New left bundle branch block
  - Previously treated like a STEMI
  - Should raise suspicion of acute event
- ST depression
  - In contiguous leads, may indicate ischemia
  - In leads V1 to V4, may indicate posterior wall injury
- Serial EKG
  - May be indicated every 15 to 30 minutes in patients who remain symptomatic in first hour after presentation

Laboratory
- Troponin
  - Negative on arrival does not rule out ischemia
  - Repeat should be done within 3 to 6 hours
  - Considered negative if no elevations 6 hours after presentation
- Complete blood count (CBC)
- Coagulation panel

Echocardiogram
- Evaluate for ejection fraction and mechanical

Stress Test
- Nuclear medicine

Treatment and Management

CLINICAL TIPS AND TRICKS

ICU VERSUS TELEMETRY ADMISSION CRITERIA

Floor
- Suspect ischemia
- Heparin infusion
- Chest pain resolved
- Low to moderate risk for NSTEMI

ICU/CCU
- Hypotension
- Unresolved chest pain
- Cardiogenic shock
- Symptomatic acute heart failure
- Systolic blood pressure (SBP) <100
- High bleed risk on heparin infusion
- Post cardiac arrest
- High risk for NSTEMI
- Electrical instability
  - Ventricular tachycardia
  - Ventricular fibrillation

- **Antiplatelet Therapy**
  - Indicated in patients with STEMI or with acute coronary syndrome (ACS) and moderate to high risk for NSTEMI
    - These patients should receive dual-platelet therapy with aspirin and another antiplatelet therapy.
  - Aspirin
    - Aspirin should be given by emergency medical services (EMSs) prior to arrival.

- ▓ If it has not be given it should be given as soon as possible after arrival to the emergency department and prior to cardiac cath lab.
- ▓ Aspirin should be continued daily in patients with acute MI or coronary disease.
- ▓ Dosages range from 81 to 325 mg daily.
- ● Clopidogrel
  - ▓ 600-mg loading dose (prior to left heart catheterization)
  - ▓ Continue at 75 mg daily in acute MI (both STEMI and NSTEMI)

OR

- ● Prasugrel
  - ▓ 60 mg loading dose (prior to left heart catheterization)

OR

- ● Ticagrelor
  - ▓ 180 mg loading dose (prior to left heart catheterization)
  - ▓ Continue at 90 mg q12h in acute MI (both STEMI and NSTEMI)
- ● Heparin
  - ▓ Bolus 50 to 70 units/kg
  - ▓ Maximum bolus 5,000 units
  - ▓ Bolus should be given prior to cardiac catheterization if possible
  - ▓ Continuous infusion after initial bolus
  - ▓ Titrated for therapeutic effect based on partial thromboplastin time (PTT)

CLINICAL TIPS AND TRICKS

HIGH-RISK INDICATORS FOR NSTEMI

- ▓ Elevated troponin
- ▓ New ST segment depression
- ▓ Angina at rest or low-stress activity while on therapy
- ▓ Ventricular tachycardia greater than 30 seconds
- ▓ Percutaneous coronary intervention (PCI) in the past 6 months

- ▓ **STATIN Therapy**
  - ● Moderate- to high-dose statin should be initiated in patients with MI and suspected MI
  - ● Dose recommended prior to PCI
  - ● Dosing should be continued on discharge
- ▓ **Nitroglycerin**
  - ● Sublingual
  - ● Intravenous
  - ● Contraindicated for hypotension

■ **Beta-Blocker**
  ● Should be given in first 24 hours and continued post discharge
  ● Decreases heart rate and blood pressure
  ● Decreases myocardial oxygen consumption
  ● Decreases risk of reinfarction
  ● Contraindication
    ■ Acute heart failure
    ■ Second- or third-degree heart block
■ **Angiotensin-Converting Enzyme (ACE) Inhibitor**
  ● Mortality benefit in acute MI with ejection fraction (EF) <40%
  ● Consider angiotensin II receptor blocker in patients unable to tolerate ACE inhibitor
  ● Patients with a history or diabetes and chronic kidney disease should be started on an ACE Inhibitor prophylactically to decrease the risk of renal failure and cardiac events.
■ **Aldosterone Antagonist**
  ● Spironolactone 25 to 25 mg daily
  ● May be beneficial in patients with acute myocardial infarction (AMI) and EF less than 40%
■ **Left Heart Catheterization and/or PCI**
  ● Indications
    ■ New ST elevation in 2 or more leads
    ■ Refractory angina
    ■ Cardiogenic shock
    ■ Ventricular tachycardia
    ■ Ventricular fibrillation
  ● Activation of cardiac catheterization lab on presentation of STEMI
  ● Goal is intervention within 90 minutes of presentation
■ **CABG**
  ● Indicated when PCI not possible
  ● Usually indicated when there is multivessel disease and stents cannot be placed.
  ● Often seen when patients have had previous stents that have failed.

Bibliography

Anderson, J. L., & Morrow, D. A. (2017). Acute myocardial infarction. *New England Journal of Medicine, 376*(21), 2053. https://doi.org/10.1056/NEJMra1606915

Bangalore, S., Makani, H., & Radford, M. (2014). Clinical outcomes with B-blockers for myocardial infarction: A meta-analysis of randomized trials. *American Journal of Medicine, 64*(24), 939–953. https://doi.org/10.1016/j.amjmed.2014.05.032

Dewilde, W. J., Oirbans, T., Verheugt, F. W. A., Kelder, J. C., De Smet, B. J. G. L., Herrman, J.-P., Adriaenssens, T., Vrolix, M., Heestermans, A. A. C. M., Vis, M. M., Tijsen, J. G.P., van 't Hof, A. W., & ten Berg, J. M.; WOEST study investigators et al. (2013). Use of clopidogrel with or without aspirin in patients taking oral

anticoagulant therapy and undergoing percutaneous coronary intervention:
An open-label randomized control trial. *Lancet, 381*, 1107–1115. https://doi.org/
10.1016/S0140-6736(12)62177-1

Hofmann, R., James, S. K., Jernberg, T., Lindahl, B., Erlinge, D., Witt, N., Arefalk,
G., Frick, M., Alfredsson, J., Nilsson, L., Ravn-Fischer, A., Omerovic, E., Kellerth,
T., Sparv, D., Ekelund, U., Linder, R., Ekström, M., Lauermann, J., Haaga, U, ...
Svensson, L. (2017). Oxygen therapy in suspected acute myocardial infarction.
The New England Journal of Medicine, 377(13), 1240–1249. https://doi.org/10.1056/
NEJMoa1706222

Maddox, T. M., Stanislawski, M. A., Grunwald, G. K., Bradley, S. M., Ho, P. M.,
Tsai, T. T., Patel, M. R., Sandhu, A., Valle, J., Magid, D. J., Leon, B., Bhatt, D. L.,
Fihn, S. D., & Rumsfeld, J. S. (2014). Nonobstructive coronary artery disease and
risk of myocardial infarction. *JAMA, 312*(17), 1744–1763. https://doi.org/10.1001/
jama.2014.14681

McCance, K. L., & Huether, S. E. (2019). *Pathophysiology: The biologic basis for disease in
adults children* (8th ed.). Mosby.

Panju, A. A., & Hemmelgarn, B. R. (1998). The rational clinical examination: Is this
patient having a myocardial infarction? *JAMA, 280*(14), 1256–1263. https://
doi.org/10.1001/jama.280.14.1256

Soliman, E. Z., Safford, M. M., Muntner, P., Khodneva, Y., Dawood, F. Z., Zakai,
N. A., Thacker, E. L., Judd, S., Howard, V. J., Howard, G., Herrington, D. M.,
& Cushman, M. (2014). Atrial fibrillation and the risk of myocardial infarction.
JAMA Internal Medicine, 174(1), E107–E114. https://doi.org/ 10.1001/
jamainternmed.2013.11912

White, H. D., & Chew, D. P. (2008). Acute myocardial infarction. *The Lancet, 372*,
570–584. https://doi.org/10.1016/S0140-6736(08)61237-4

2

HYPERTENSION URGENCY AND EMERGENCY

CLINICAL TIPS AND TRICKS

HYPERTENSIVE URGENCY VERSUS HYPERTENSIVE EMERGENCY
Hypertensive Urgency

Extreme asymptomatic hypertension, with no signs of end-organ damage

Hypertensive Emergency

Severe hypertension with signs and symptoms of end-organ damage

HYPERTENSIVE URGENCY

Cause

- Refractory hypertension
- Medication noncompliance

Risk Factors

- Obesity
- Tobacco use
- Excessive alcohol consumption
- Estrogen supplementation
- Pregnancy
- Endocrine disorders
  - Pheochromocytoma

Assessment Findings

- Systolic blood pressure (SBP) >170 or diastolic blood pressure (DBP) >110
- May be asymptomatic with only finding being elevated BP
- Headache but overall asymptomatic

Diagnostics

Laboratory
- Troponin
  - Evaluate for cardiac damage
- Serum chemistry
  - Evaluate renal function

Treatment and Management

- **Medication**
  - Intravenous (IV) medication is not usually indicated in asymptomatic patients
  - Clonidine PO 0.1 to 0.2 mg
  - Captopril 6.25 to 12.5 mg
- Patient may not need admission if no other symptom noted
- BP should be lowered over hours or days
- Will need primary care follow-up
- May be managed as an outpatient if patient is otherwise stable
- **Goal BP: SBP <160, DBP <110**
  - Be aware to not lower BP too low or too quick

HYPERTENSIVE EMERGENCY

Cause

- Refractory hypertension
- Medication noncompliance
- Aortic dissection
- Stroke
- Pulmonary edema
- Malignant hypertension
- Preeclampsia or eclampsia
- Intracranial hemorrhage
- Myocardial infarction
- Pheochromocytoma
- Drug intoxication
  - Cocaine
  - Amphetamines

CLINICAL TIPS AND TRICKS

AORTIC DISSECTION
- Severe sudden pain
  - Back pain
  - Chest pain
- Hypertension
  - Seen with descending aorta dissection
- Hypotension
  - Seen with ascending aorta dissection
- Weakened pulses
  - Carotid
  - Brachial
  - Femoral
- Syncope
- Diastolic decrescendo murmur
- Wide pulse pressure
- Widen mediastinum on chest x-ray

Assessment Findings

Cardiovascular
- SBP >180 or DBP >110 to 120
  - No set standard
- Tachycardia
- Bradycardia
- Jugular vein distention (JVD)
- Chest pain

Neurological
- Blurred vision or vision loss
- Agitation
- Stupor
- Delirium
- Headache
- Lethargy
- Seizures
- Nausea and vomiting
  - Can be a sign of increased intracranial pressure

Fundoscopic Exam
- Should be performed on any patient in whom hypertensive crisis is suspected
- Optic disk edema
- Flame hemorrhages
- Cotton wool spots

CLINICAL TIPS AND TRICKS

FUNDOSCOPIC EXAM IN HYPERTENSION

Papilledema: Swelling of the optic disk

Cotton Wool Spots: White spots or patches on the retina

Flame Hemorrhages: Flame-shaped hemorrhages caused by necrotic vessels that bleed into the superficial capillary beds

Back Pain
- Specific to aortic dissection

Pulmonary
- Dyspnea

Diagnostics

Laboratory
- Serum chemistry panel
  - Elevated BUN
  - Elevated creatinine
- Serum lactate
  - Elevation indicates hypoperfusion
- Troponin
- Urinalysis
- Urine or serum drug screen
  - When substance abuse is the suspected cause

Radiography
- Chest radiography
- Head CT
  - When concerns for intracranial process such as the following:
    - Acute cerebrovascular accident (CVA)
    - Intracranial hemorrhage
    - Recent head trauma
- Chest CT
  - Suspected aortic dissection

EKG
- Consider in all significantly hypertensive patients for concerns of ischemia or acute myocardial infarction

Treatment and Management

CLINICAL TIPS AND TRICKS

COCAINE-INDUCED HYPERTENSIVE EMERGENCY

- Beta-blockers are contraindicated in treatment of cocaine-induced hypertension
- Treatment includes the following:
  - Alpha-blockers
  - Benzodiazepines
  - Calcium channel blocker infusion
  - Clonidine

- **Arterial line placement**
  - Allows for continuous hemodynamic monitoring
- **Requires critical care management**
  - ICU- or CCU-level admission
- **BP should be lowered gradually**
  - Initial SBP goal 160 to 180 mmHg
  - Initial DBP goal 90 to 100 mmHg
  - Goals specific to patient
- **Medication options**
  - Nicardipine
    - 5 mg/hr with maximum of 15 mg/hr
  - Nitroglycerin
    - 0.5 to 10 mcg/kg/min
    - 5 to 100 mcg/min
    - Helpful in heart failure and ischemia
    - Decreases preload and some afterload
  - Nitroprusside
    - 1 to 10 mcg/kg/min
    - May cause rapid decrease in BP
    - Not recommended for use for greater than 72 hours due to risk of cyanide toxicity
    - Has significant afterload reduction
  - Labetalol
    - 20 to 40 mg q10min
    - Up to 2 mg/min continuous infusion

- Hydralazine
  - 5 to 20 mg IV push
  - Not used in aortic dissection
- Esmolol
  - Loading dose of 500 to 1,000 mcg
  - 25 to 50 mcg/kg/min with maximum of 300 mcg/kg/min
  - May cause significant bradycardia
- Enalapril
  - 1.25 mg over 5 minutes q6h
- **Cardiac catheterization**
  - Consider if ischemia is suspected
- **Other underlying conditions**
  - Identify underlying conditions that may exist
  - Treatment for underlying condition as indicated by the system

Bibliography

Jamerson, K., Weber, M. A., Bakris, G. L., Dahlöf, B., Pitt, B., Shi, V., Hester, A., Gupte, J., Gatlin, M., & Velazquez, E. J.; ACCOMPLISH Trial Investigators (2008). Benazepril plus amlodipine or hydrochlorothiazide for hypertension in high-risk patients. *New England Journal of Medicine, 359*(23), 2417. https://doi.org/10.1056/NEJMoa0806182

Karabacak, M., Yiquit, M., Turdogan, K. A., & Sert, M. (2015). The relationship between vascular inflammation and target organ damage in hypertensive crises. *American Journal of Emergency Medicine, 33*(4), 497–500. https://doi.org/10.1016/j.ajem.2014.11.014.

McCance, K. L., & Huether, S. E. (2019). *Pathophysiology: The biologic basis for disease in adults children* (8th ed.). Mosby.

Preston R. A., Arciniegas, R., DeGraff, S., Materson, B. J., Bernstein, J., & Afshartous, D. (2019). Outcomes of minority patients with very severe hypertension (>220/>120 mmHg). *Journal of Hypertension, 37*(2), 415. https://doi.org/10.1097/HJH.0000000000001906

Varon, K. (2000). The diagnosis and management of hypertensive crises. *Chest, 118*(1), 214–227. https://doi.org/10.1378/chest.118.1.214

Varon, K. (2008). Treatment of acute severe hypertension: Current and newer agents. *Drugs, 68*(3), 283–297. https://doi.org/10.2165/00003495-200868030-00003

Whelton, P. K., Carey, R. M., Aronow, W. S., Casey, D. E., Jr., Collins, K. J., Himmelfarb, C. D., DePalma, S. M., Gidding, S., Jamerson, K. A., Jones, D. W., MacLaughlin, E. J., Muntner, P., Ovbiagele, B., Smith, S. C., Jr., Spencer, C. C., Stafford, R. S., Taler, S. J., Thomas, R. J., Williams, K. A., Sr., ... Wright, J. T., Jr. (2018). 2017 ACC/AHA/AAPA/ABC/ACPM/AGS/APhA/ASH/ASPC/NMA/PCNA guideline for the prevention, detection, evaluation, and management of high blood pressure in adults: A report of the American College of Cardiology/American Heart Association Task Force on Clinical Practice Guidelines. *Hypertension, 71*(6), e13. https://doi.org/10.1161/HYP.0000000000000065

Wong, T. Y., & Mitchell, P. (2007). The eye in hypertension. *Lancet, 369*, 425. https://doi.org/10.1016/S0140-6736(07)60198-6

3

MANAGEMENT OF ACUTE HEART FAILURE

HEART FAILURE WITH REDUCED EJECTION FRACTION

Causes

Left Ventricular Systolic Dysfunction

- Coronary artery disease
- Idiopathic dilated cardiomyopathy
- Muscular dystrophy
- Alcohol abuse
- Cocaine abuse
- Myocarditis
- Peripartum
- Untreated valvular heart disease
- Tachyarrhythmias
- Hypertension
- Lupus
- Rheumatoid arthritis

CLINICAL TIPS AND TRICKS

NEW YORK HEART ASSOCIATION FUNCTIONAL CLASSIFICATION

I = No symptoms
II = Symptoms with moderate or marked levels of activity
III = Symptoms with mild activity
IV = Symptoms at rest

Assessment Findings

General

- Cool extremities
- Altered mentation

Cardiovascular

- Tachycardia
- Jugular venous distention
- Hepatojugular reflux
- Narrow pulse pressure

- Hypotension
- S3 and/or S4
- Tricuspid murmur

Pulmonary
- Shortness of breath
- Cheyne–Stokes respirations
- Rales

Diagnostics

Laboratory
- Serum chemistries
- Complete blood count (CBC)
- Troponin
- Brain natriuretic peptide (BNP)
  - May be useful in patients in whom cause of dyspnea is not known

Radiology
- Chest x-ray

EKG

Echocardiogram
- Especially important in a patient with an unknown ejection fraction (EF) or first presentation of decompensated heart failure

Treatment and Management

Admission Decision
- *Telemetry*
  - Minimum standard for exacerbation of heart failure
  - Stable vital signs
  - No continuous infusions of diuretic
  - Blood pressure controlled
- *Step down*
  - Depends on the ability of the facility
  - Patient requires higher level of monitoring but not critical
- *ICU*
  - Patient unstable
  - Shock present
  - Mechanical ventilation
  - Continuous diuretic infusion
  - Non-invasive ventilation
  - Inotropic medications

Respiratory Support
- Assess ventilation and work of breathing
- Supplemental oxygen for hypoxia

- ▓ Bipap
  - ● Help with increased work of breathing
  - ● Improve ventilation
- ▓ Intubation/mechanical ventilation
  - ● For respiratory failure

Medications
- ▓ Bolus dose loop diuretics
  - ● Requires close monitoring of input/output (I/O)
  - ● Consider Foley catheter for accurate assessment of volume status
  - ● Especially important in incontinent patients or critically ill patient's
  - ● patients on a diuretic infusion should have catheter in place for hourly I&O
  - ● Furosemide
    - ▓ Initial dose 40 to 60 mg or double home dose
    - ▓ Maximum daily dose 160 to 320 mg
  - ● Bumetanide
    - ▓ Initial dose 1 to 2 mg
    - ▓ Maximum dose 5 to 10 mg
- ▓ Continuous infusion loop diuretics
  - ● Requires close monitoring of electrolytes
  - ● Monitor closely for symptoms of hypokalemia
  - ● Requires foley catheter placement
  - ● Furosemide
    - ▓ 20 to 80 mg loading dose
    - ▓ 5 to 20 mg/hr
  - ● Bumetanide
    - ▓ 1 mg IV load
    - ▓ 0.5 to 2 mg/hr
- ▓ Morphine
  - ● Assists with air hunger
- ▓ Nitrates
  - ● Nitroglycerin
    - ▓ 5 to 25 mcg/min
    - ▓ max 300 mcg/min
    - ▓ Coronary vasodilators
    - ▓ Decreases systemic pressure
    - ▓ Decreases pulmonary pressure
  - ● Nitroprusside
    - ▓ 0.5 to 8 mcg/kg/min
    - ▓ max 10 mcg/kg min
    - ▓ Extremely potent and can cause extreme hypotension
    - ▓ Use with caution and titrate carefully
    - ▓ Should be used with arterial line monitoring only
    - ▓ Nitroprusside is only used for max 72 hours as it can metabolize into cyanide
    - ▓ Decreases preload and afterload

- Inotropes
  - Used in patients with known depressed ejection fraction or cardiogenic shock.
  - Used to improve cardiac output and cardiac index.
  - Recommend advanced hemodynamic monitoring to assist with titration.
    - Dobutamine
      - 2.5 to 20 mcg/kg/min
      - max dose 40 mcg/kg/min
    - Milrinone
      - Initial bolus 50 mcg/kg over 10 min
      - 0.375 to 0.75 mcg/kg/min

Follow-Up
- Intracardiac defibrillators (ICDs)
  - Recommended in patients with EF <30% due to increased risk of sudden cardiac death
  - Some patients may have Life Vest placed initially if ICD cannot be implanted or are expected to have improvement in EF

HEART FAILURE WITH PRESERVED EJECTION FRACTION

Causes

- Infiltrative heart disease
- Constrictive pericarditis
- Hypertension
- Anemia
- Thyrotoxicosis
- Arteriovenous (AV) communication
- Obesity
- Right-side heart failure from pulmonary disease

Assessment Findings

General
- Cool extremities
- Altered mentation

Cardiovascular
- Tachycardia
- Jugular venous distention
- Hepatojugular reflux
- Narrow pulse pressure
- Hypotension
- S3 and/or S4
- Tricuspid murmur

Pulmonary
- Shortness of breath
- Cheyne–Stokes respirations
- Rales

Diagnostics

Laboratory
- Serum chemistries
- CBC
- Troponin
- BNP
  - May be useful in patients in whom cause of dyspnea is not known

Radiology
- Chest x-ray

EKG

Echocardiogram

Treatment and Management

Admission Decision
- Telemetry
  - Minimum standard for exacerbation of heart failure
  - Stable vital signs
  - No continuous infusions of diuretic
  - Blood pressure controlled
- Step down
  - Depends on facility
  - Patient requires higher level of monitoring but not critical
- ICU
  - Patient hemodynamically unstable
  - Shock present
  - Mechanical ventilation
  - Non-invasive ventilation
  - Vasopressors
  - Diuretic infusion

Respiratory Support
- Assess ventilation and work of breathing
- Supplemental oxygen for hypoxia
- Bipap
  - Help with increased work of breathing
  - Improve ventilation
- Intubation/mechanical ventilation
  - For respiratory failure

CLINICAL TIPS AND TRICKS

MEDICATIONS
Diuretic Infusions

■ Foley catheter highly recommended for accurate I/O
■ Frequent monitoring of electrolytes (every 4–6 hours)
■ Replacement of potassium and other electrolytes
■ Set 24-hr goal for net urine output

■ Bolus dose loop diuretics
  ● Furosemide
    ■ Initial dose 40 to 60 mg or double home dose
    ■ Maximum daily dose 160 to 320 mg
  ● Bumetanide
    ■ Initial dose 1 to 2 mg
    ■ Maximum dose 5 to 10 mg
■ Continuous infusion loop diuretics
  ● Furosemide
    ■ 20 to 80 mg loading dose
    ■ 5 to 20 mg/hr
  ● Bumetanide
    ■ 1 mg IV load
    ■ 0.5 to 2 mg/hr
■ Morphine
  ● Assists with air hunger
■ Nitroglycerin
  ● 5 to 25 mcg/min
  ● max 300 mcg/min
  ● Coronary vasodilators
  ● Decrease systemic pressure
  ● Decrease pulmonary pressure
■ Nitroprusside
  ● 0.5 to 8 mcg/kg/min
  ● max 10 mcg/kg min
  ● Decreases preload and afterload

Bibliography

Maddox, T. M., Stanislawski, M. A., Grunwald, G. K., Bradley, S. M., Ho, P. M., Tsai, T. T., Patel, M. R., Sandhu, A., Valle, J., Magid, D. J., Leon, B., Bhatt, D. L., Fihn, S. D., & Rumsfeld, J. S. (2014). Nonobstructive coronary artery disease and risk of myocardial infarction. *JAMA, 312*(17), 1744–1763. https://doi.org/10.1001/jama.2014.14681
McCance, K. L., & Huether, S. E. (2019). *Pathophysiology: The biologic basis for disease in adults children* (8th ed.). Mosby.

Ponikowski, P. (2016). 2016 ESC guidelines for the diagnosis and treatment of acute and chronic heart failure: The Task Force for the diagnosis and treatment of acute and chronic heart failure of the European Society of Cardiology (ESC) developed with the special contribution of the Heart Failure Association (HFA) of the ESC. *European Heart Journal, 37*(27), 2129. https://doi.org/10.1093/eurheartj/ehw128

Preston R. A., Arciniegas, R., DeGraff, S., Materson, B. J., Bernstein, J., & Afshartous, D. (2019). Outcomes of minority patients with very severe hypertension (>220/>120 mmHg). *Journal of Hypertension, 37*(2), 415. https://doi.org/10.1097/HJH.0000000000001906

Whelton, P. K., Carey, R. M., Carey, R. M., Aronow, W. S., Casey, D. E., Jr., Collins, K. J., Himmelfarb, C. D., DePalma, S. M., Gidding, S., Jamerson, K. A., Jones, D. W., MacLaughlin, E. J., Muntner, P., Ovbiagele, B., Smith, S. C., Jr., Spencer, C. C., Stafford, R. S., Taler, S. J., Thomas, R. J., Williams, K. A., Sr., ... Wright, J. T., Jr. (2018). 2017 ACC/AHA/AAPA/ABC/ACPM/AGS/APhA/ASH/ASPC/NMA/PCNA guideline for the prevention, detection, evaluation, and management of high blood pressure in adults: A report of the American College of Cardiology/American Heart Association Task Force on Clinical Practice Guidelines. *Hypertension, 71*(6), e13. https://doi.org/10.1161/HYP.0000000000000065

Yancy, C. W., Januzzi, J. L., Jr., Allen, L. A., Butler, J., Davis, L. L., Fonarow, G. C., Ibrahim, N. E., Jessup, M., Lindenfeld, J., Maddox, T. M., Masoudi, F. A., Motiwala, S. R., Patterson, J. H., Walsh, M. N., & Wasserman, A. (2017). ACC expert consensus decision pathway for optimization of heart failure treatment: Answers to 10 pivotal issues about heart failure with reduced ejection fraction: A report of the American College of Cardiology Task Force on expert consensus decision pathways. *Journal of the American College of Cardiology, 71*(2), 201. https://doi.org/10.1016/j.jacc.2017.11.025

SECTION II

PULMONARY DISORDERS AND MANAGEMENT

4

RESPIRATORY FAILURE

Causes

Neurological
- Change in level of consciousness
  - Opiate overdose
- Neuromuscular disease
  - Guillain–Barré syndrome
  - Myasthenia gravis
- Spinal cord injury

Chest
- Trauma to chest wall
- Obesity
- Kyphosis
- Pneumothorax
- Hemothorax
- Abdominal distention
- Pleural effusion

Lung parenchyma
- Edema
- Atelectasis
- Infiltrate

Airway
- Upper airway
  - Tumor
  - Edema
    - Allergic reaction
    - Angioedema
  - Foreign body
  - Abscess
  - Trauma
- Lower airway
  - Foreign body
  - Mucus plug
  - Tumor
  - Bronchospasm

Vascular
- Pulmonary embolism
- Right ventricular failure

CLINICAL TIPS AND TRICKS

SHUNT AND DEAD SPACE
Shunt
A shunt is when blood is not oxygenated. There are two types: physiological and anatomic.
Physiological Shunt
Most common type of shunt. This happens when perfusion is inadequate due to collapsed alveoli.
Anatomic Shunt
Physical diversion of blood that bypasses the lungs for oxygenation. Patent foramen ovale or septal defect can be a common cause of anatomic shunt.
Dead Space
Area of lung that has inadequate perfusion or decreases alveolar lung surface.

Assessment Findings

General
- Altered mental status
- Decreased level of consciousness
- Anxiety
- Diaphoresis
- Cyanosis

Respiratory
- Increased work of breathing
- Tachypnea
- Hypoxia
- Ancillary muscle use
- Abnormal lung sounds
  - Dependent of pathology
- Mucus production
- Cough

Cardiovascular
- Tachycardia
- Bradycardia
  - Sign of severe hypoxia
- Hypotension/shock

Diagnostics

Laboratory
- Arterial blood gas
- Complete blood count (CBC)
- Chemistries
- Lactic

Radiology

CLINICAL TIPS AND TRICKS

CHEST X-RAY READING TIPS

A—Airway
- Ensure trachea is midline
- Check for a widened mediastinum

B—Bones
- Check for fractures
- Check for dislocations
- Spine and humerus including osteoarthritic changes
- Soft tissues for subcutaneous air, foreign bodies, and surgical clips

C—Cardiac
- Check heart size and heart borders
  - Appropriate or blunted
  - Thin rim of air around the heart, think of pneumomediastinum
- Check aorta
  - Widening, tortuosity, calcification
- Check heart valves
  - Calcification, valve replacements
- Check superior vena cava (SVC), inferior vena cava (IVC)
  - Widening, tortuosity

D—Diaphragm
- Right hemidiaphragm
  - Should be higher than the left
  - If much higher, think of effusion, lobar collapse, diaphragmatic paralysis
  - If you cannot see parts of the diaphragm, consider infiltrate or effusion

E—Effusion
- Effusions
  - Look for blunting of the costophrenic angle.
  - Identify the major fissures; if you can see them more obvious than usual, then this could mean that fluid is tracking along the fissure.
- Evaluate pleura
  - Thickening, loculations, calcifications, and pneumothorax

---

(continued)

F—Fields
- Infiltrates
  - Identify the location of infiltrates by use of known radiological phenomena, for example, loss of heart borders or of the contour of the diaphragm.
  - Remember that right middle lobe abuts the heart, but the right lower lobe does not.
  - The lingula abuts the left side of the heart.
- Identify the pattern of infiltration
  - Interstitial pattern (reticular) versus alveolar (patchy or nodular) pattern
  - Lobar collapse
  - Look for air bronchograms, tram tracking, nodules, Kerley B lines
  - Pay attention to the apices
- Look for granulomas, tumor, and pneumothorax

G—Gastric Air Bubble
- Check correct position
- Beware of hiatus hernia
- Look for free air
- Look for bowel loops between diaphragm and liver

H—Hilum
- Check the position and size bilaterally
- Enlarged lymph nodes
- Calcified nodules
- Mass lesions
- Pulmonary arteries; if greater than 1.5 cm, think about possible causes of enlargement

- **Chest x-ray**
  - Anterior–posterior (AP)
  - Posterior–anterior (PA) and lateral
- **EKG**
- **Bronchoscopy**
  - Diagnostics
    - Evaluation of disease
    - Evaluate structures and mucosa
    - Take biopsies
  - Therapeutic
    - Removal of secretions
    - Removal of foreign bodies
    - Removal of mucous plugging

Treatment and Management

CLINICAL TIPS AND TRICKS

INTUBATION CRITERIA
Degree of distress

- Evaluate degree of distress
- Respiratory rate >30
- Work of breathing
- Ancillary muscle use
- Apnea
- Age and ability to sustain level of distress

Gas exchange

- Evaluation of arterial blood gas
- Hypoxemia
- Ventilation
- Acidosis with pH <7.25

Progression of underlying process

- How long will it take to correct the underlying condition?
- Can patient maintain airway until the condition is corrected?
- Level of consciousness
- Hemodynamic instability

Noninvasive Ventilation
- Continuous positive airway pressure
- Bilevel positive airway pressure (BiPAP)
- May be beneficial in patients who do not require more than 48 hours of support and can protect their airway

Mechanical Ventilation
- Goals
  - Improve ventilation
    - Minute ventilation (MV) = tidal volume × respiratory rate
    - Manipulate respiratory rate
      - Increasing respiratory rate will decrease CO_2
      - Increasing respiratory rate will increase MV

- ■ Manipulate tidal volume
  - ● Increasing tidal volume will decrease CO_2
  - ● Increasing respiratory rate will increase MV
- ● Improve oxygenation
  - ■ Increase in positive end-expiratory pressure (PEEP) can improve oxygenation
  - ■ Increasing MV may increase oxygenation
- ■ Treat underlying cause
  - ● These can vary widely, from neurological to respiratory in origin

BIBLIOGRAPHY

Adler, D., Pépin, J.-L., Dupuis-Lozeron, E., Espa-Cervena, K., Merlet-Violet, R., Muller, H., Janssens, J.-P., & Brochard, L. (2017). Comorbidities and subgroups of patients surviving severe acute hypercapnic respiratory failure in the intensive care unit. *American Journal of Respiratory and Critical Care Medicine, 196*(2), 200. https://doi.org/10.1164/rccm.201608-1666OC

McCance, K. L., & Huether, S. E. (2019). *Pathophysiology: The biologic basis for disease in adults children* (8th ed.). Mosby.

Ram, F. S., Picot, J., Lightowler, J., & Wedzicha J. A. (2004). Non-invasive positive pressure ventilation for treatment of respiratory failure due to exacerbations of chronic obstructive pulmonary disease. *The Cochrane Database of Systematic Reviews*, (1), CD004104. https://doi.org/10.1002/14651858.CD004104.pub2

Tobin, M. J., Jubran, A., & Laghi, F. (2001). Patient-ventilator interaction. *American Journal of Respiratory Critical Care Medicine, 163*(5), 1059. https://doi.org/10.1164/ajrccm.163.5.2005125

Wilson, J. G., & Matthay, M. A. (2014). Mechanical Ventilation in acute hypoxemic respiratory failure: A review of new strategies for the practicing hospitalist. *Journal of Hospital Medicine, 9*(7), 469–475. https://doi.org/10.1002/jhm.2192

ADULT RESPIRATORY DISTRESS SYNDROME

Causes

- Sepsis
- Pneumonia
  - Aspiration pneumonia
- Blunt force trauma
- Fat embolism
- Transfusion-related acute lung injury (TRALI)
  - Adult respiratory distress syndrome (ARDS) that develops after transfusion of blood products
- Massive blood transfusion
  - Required in trauma or massive hemorrhage

CLINICAL TIPS AND TRICKS

STAGES OF ADULT RESPIRATORY DISTRESS SYNDROME
Exudative Phase

- Occurs between days 5 and 7
- Systemic inflammation
- Increased permeability of alveolar–capillary barrier
- Leads to pulmonary edema
- Extravasation of neutrophils migrates leading to alveolar hemorrhage

Proliferative Phase

- Occurs between days 7 and 21
- **Fibrotic changes begin to occur**

Fibrotic Phase

- Occurs after several weeks of development
- Possible long-term pulmonary fibrosis

Assessment Findings

General
- Fever
- Hemodynamic instability
- Symptoms of underlying condition such as sepsis or trauma
- Cyanosis

Respiratory
- Dyspnea
- Cough
- Sudden increase in oxygen requirement
- Hypoxia
- Sputum production
- Elevated peak airway pressures
- Paradoxical breathing
- Abnormal lung sounds
  - Wheezing
  - Rhonchi
  - Stridor

Cardiovascular
- Tachycardia
- Hypotension
- Shock symptoms

Neurological
- Confusion
- Altered mental status
- Decreased level of consciousness
- Restlessness

Diagnostics

Lab
- Complete blood count (CBC)
- Serum chemistry
- D-dimer
- Brain natriuretic peptide (BNP)
- Arterial blood gas

CLINICAL TIPS AND TRICKS

P/F RATIO CALCULATIONS

$PaO_2/FiO_2 = P/F$ ratio
Example: PaO_2 is 70 and FiO_2 is 70%
$P/F = 100$
FiO_2 used as a decimal; 70% becomes 0.70

Radiology
■ **Chest x-ray**
  ● Findings
    ■ Bilateral diffuse opacities
    ■ Ground glass opacities
    ■ "White out" chest x-ray
■ **Chest CT**
  ● May be helpful to determine the extent of ARDS

Microbiology
■ Sputum culture
■ Bronchoscopy cultures

Echocardiogram
■ Helpful in determining cardiogenic pulmonary edema versus ARDS

CLINICAL TIPS AND TRICKS

ADULT RESPIRATORY DISTRESS SYNDROME SEVERITY

Mild ARDS P/F ratio
200 to 300 mmHg
Moderate ARDS P/F ratio
100 to 200 mmHg
Severe ARDS P/F ratio
<100 mmHg

Treatment and Management

Low Tidal Volume Ventilation Strategy
■ Recommend volumes of 6 to 8 mL per kg of ideal body weight.
■ Low tidal volume strategies have been shown to be lung protective in ARDS.
■ Ideal body weight should be calculated in obese patients.

Permissive Hypercapnia
■ With low tidal volume, a moderate level of hypercapnia is tolerated.

Fluid Management
■ Fluids should be optimal for the situation.
■ Fluid restriction may be beneficial in helping with pulmonary edema.
■ Diuresis should be used for volume overload.

Sedation
■ Optimizing sedation may decrease oxygenation consumption during critical illness.
■ Daily sedation holidays should still be performed to assess patient neurological status and avoid sedation build-up.

Prone Positioning
■ Improvement in oxygenation when used consistently

- Prone goals of 18 to 22 hours per day
- Prone position for at least 16 hours per day

Neuromuscular Blockade
- May improve patient-ventilator synchrony
- Generally used in early stages of ARDS

ECMO
- Not appropriate in all instances
- No mortality benefit
- Should only be used in patients with reversible injury

Inhaled Nitric Oxide
- Shows improvement of oxygenation
- No significant mortality benefit

High-Frequency Oscillatory Ventilation
- Early introduction may increase mortality
- May be appropriate in patients with severe refractory hypoxia
- No mortality benefit

Treat Underlying Cause
- Antibiotics
  - Sepsis
  - Pneumonia
  - Aspiration pneumonia
- Bronchodilators
  - Albuterol
  - Levalbuterol
- Steroids
  - No ideal time
  - Controversial; some studies suggest an increase in mortality

Bibliography

Brodie, D., & Bacchetta, M. (2011). Extracorporeal membrane oxygenation for ARDS in adults. *New England Journal of Medicine, 365*(20), 1905–1914. https://doi.org/10.1056/NEJMct1103720

Cheng, I. W., Eisner, M. D., Thompson, B. T., Ware, L. B., & Matthay, M. A. (2005). Acute effects of tidal volume strategy on hemodynamics, fluid balance, and sedation in acute lung injury. *Critical Care Medicine, 33*(1), 63. https://doi.org/10.1097/01.ccm.0000149836.76063.71

Chimello, D., & Brioni, M. (2016). Severe hypoxemia: Which strategy to choose. *Critical Care, 20*(1), 132. https://ccforum.biomedcentral.com/track/pdf/10.1186/s13054-016-1304-7.pdf

Fan, E., Brodie, D., & Slutsky, A. S. (2018). Acute respiratory distress syndrome: Advances in diagnosis and treatment. *JAMA, 319*(7), 698–710. https://doi.org/10.1001/jama.2017.21907

McCance, K. L., & Huether, S. E. (2019). *Pathophysiology: The biologic basis for disease in adults children* (8th ed.). Mosby.

Tobin, M. J., Jubran, A., & Laghi, F. (2001). Patient-ventilator interaction. *American Journal of Respiratory Critical Care Medicine, 163*(5), 1059. https://doi.org/10.1164/ajrccm.163.5.2005125

Wilson, J. G., & Matthay, M. A. (2014). Mechanical ventilation in acute hypoxemic respiratory failure: A review of new strategies for the practicing hospitalist. *Journal of Hospital Medicine, 9*(7), 469–475. https://doi.org/10.1002/jhm.2192

Yonsuck, K. (2014). Update in acute respiratory distress syndrome. *Journal of Intensive Care, 2*(2), 1–6. https://doi.org/10.1186/2052-0492-2-2

Zambon, M., & Vincent, J. L. (2008). Mortality rates for patients with acute lung injury/ARDS have decreased over time. *Chest, 133*(5), 1120. https://doi.org/10.1378/chest.07-2134

MANAGEMENT OF NEUROLOGICAL CONDITIONS

6

TRANSISCHEMIC ATTACKS AND CEREBROVASCULAR ACCIDENTS

TRANSISCHEMIC ATTACKS

Causes

Embolic
- Particles of debris that originate elsewhere in the body block blood flow to a region of the brain

Thrombosis
- Manual obstruction of an artery due to disease of the artery wall or fibromuscular dysplasia

Lacunar or Small Vessel
- Disease of the small vessels of the brain that may decrease microperfusion to the brain

Low Flow
- Due to low blood flow of stenosed vessels in the brain

Systemic Hypoperfusion
- Due to low blood flow to the brain; may be seen in systemic hemorrhage or heart failure

CLINICAL TIPS AND TRICKS

TRANSISCHEMIC ATTACK FACTS
- Can be a sign of impending cerebrovascular accident (CVA)
- Underrecognized
- Neurological emergency
- Can result in permanent ischemic tissue injury
- Most events resolve in 30 to 60 minutes
- Focus should be on symptoms

Assessment Findings

- Sudden onset of symptoms
- Hemiparesis
- Dysarthria
- Dysphasia
- Diplopia
- Circumoral numbness
- Imbalance
- Monocular blindness

Diagnostics

Radiology
- CT head
  - Imaging can be normal or show chronic changes
- MRI brain
  - May show areas of ischemia better than CT
  - May still be negative
- Magnetic resonance angiography (MRA) head
  - May show occlusion or vascular

Ultrasound
- Carotid artery dopplers
  - Evaluate for plaque or occlusion

Echocardiograph
- Bubble study
  - Evaluate for septal defect

Treatment and Management

- Evaluate risk of future stroke
- Hospitalization generally indicated for 24 hours
- Adequate blood pressure control
- Lifestyle changes
  - Tobacco cessation
  - Weight loss
- Good glycemic control

CEREBROVASCULAR ACCIDENTS

Causes

Vascular Disorders
- Atherosclerosis
  - Disease in the brain and neck
  - Most common cause in older adults
- Carotid or vertebral artery dissection

- Fibromuscular dysplasia
  - Common cause in younger adults
- Giant cell arteritis
- Systemic lupus erythematosus
- Cocaine use
  - Can cause cerebral vasospasm
  - Rupture arteriovenous (AV) malformations
- Moyamoya syndrome
- Dissection of carotid or vertebral arteries

Embolism
- Atrial fibrillation
- Atrial flutter
- Mitral or aortic valve disease
- Carotid artery arteriosclerosis
- Sickle cell disease
- Prosthetic heart valves
- Rheumatic heart disease
- Bacterial endocarditis
  - Commonly seen in intravenous (IV) drug users
- Atrial septal defect
- Atrial myxoma

Hypercoagulable States
- Antiphospholipid antibody syndrome
- Oral contraceptives
- Polycythemia
- Sickle cell disease
- Leukemia
- Activated protein C resistance
- Protein C, S, or antithrombin III deficiency
- Disseminated intravascular coagulopathy

Systemic Hypoperfusion
- Heart failure with ejection fraction <30%

CLINICAL TIPS AND TRICKS

RISK FACTORS FOR ATHEROSCLEROSIS
- Hypertension
- Tobacco use
- Hyperlipidemia
- Diabetes
- Mitral valve disease

(continued)

- Anterior wall myocardial infarction (MI)
- Advanced age
- Alcohol abuse
- Drug abuse

Assessment Findings

General
- Sudden onset of symptoms
- Hemiparesis
- Dysarthria
- Dysphasia
- Diplopia
- Circumoral numbness
- Imbalance
- Monocular blindness
- Carotid bruits

Middle Cerebral Artery Occlusion
- Hemiplegia
- Blindness of half vision field
- Aphasia

Anterior Cerebral Artery Occlusion
- Hemiplegia
  - Generally affects the lower extremities
- Urinary incontinence
- Behavior changes
- Return of primitive reflexes

Vertebral and Basilary Arteries Occlusion
- Sensory and motor deficits
- Ipsilateral cranial nerve findings

Subarachnoid Hemorrhage
- Sudden intense headache
- May radiate to posterior neck; worsened by neck movement

Intracranial Hemorrhage
- Hypertension
- Headache
- Eye deviation
  - Conjugately
  - Downward

- Pinpoint pupils
- Coma
- Vertigo

Diagnostics

Radiology
- CT head
  - Lacunar infarct
    - Degenerative changes from small arteries deep in the brain
  - Assessment for intracranial bleeding prior to the administration of tissue plasminogen activator (tPA)
  - Will differentiate between ischemic and hemorrhagic stroke
- MRI brain
  - More sensitive than CT
  - May show ischemia
- MRA head
  - Evaluation of intracranial vessels and extracranial vessels

Ultrasound
- Carotid artery dopplers
- Evaluate for carotid artery occlusion

Echocardiograph
- Bubble study
  - Evaluate for atrio-septal defect

Laboratory
- Chemistry
  - Hypoglycemia can mimic stroke symptoms
  - Electrolyte abnormalities
- Coagulation panel
  - Evaluate for coagulopathy
  - Baseline prior to initiating anticoagulation therapy
- Lipid panel
- Eosinophil sedimentary rate (ESR)
  - Elevated in vasculitis, endocarditis, giant cell arteritis

Microbiology
- Blood cultures
  - Evaluate for endocarditis

EKG
- Identify atrial fibrillation or atrial flutter.

Treatment and Management

CLINICAL TIPS AND TRICKS

TISSUE PLASMINOGEN ACTIVATOR GUIDELINES*
Exclusion Criteria
- Used for ischemic strokes
- Last known baseline within 4.5 hours of administration
- Systolic blood pressure (SBP) <180 mmHg
- Diastolic blood pressure (DBP) <110 mmHg
- Platelets <100,000
- No signs of acute bleeding
- Age >18 years
- No intracranial malignancy
- No previous CVA in 3 months prior to current event
- No head trauma in previous 3 months
- No history of recent gastrointestinal (GI) bleed

High-Risk Warnings
- Recent serious trauma
- Recent major surgery
- Remote history of GI bleeding
- Recent arterial puncture
- Large intracranial aneurysm
- Age >80 years
- Pregnancy

*Need accurate body weight prior to dosing

Blood Pressure Control
- If patient is hypertensive, control blood pressure
- Avoid hypotension
- Goal is 140 to 160 seconds for optimum perfusion pressure
  - Based on patient clinical appearance
- See Chapter 2 for management tips

Diabetes
- Adequate glucose management in patients with diabetes

Fibrinolytic Therapy
- Alteplase
  - See Clinical Tips and Tricks (Tissue Plasminogen Activator Guidelines)
  - Evaluate bleeding risk

Mechanical Thrombectomy
- Done for large artery occlusions
- Can be done up to 24 hours from the last known neurological baseline
- Can be performed even if the patient has received thrombolytics

Subarachnoid Hemorrhage
- Continuous cardiac monitoring
- Reversal of anticoagulation medications
- Monitoring for cerebral edema and increase in intracranial pressure (ICP)
- Neurosurgery consult is generally indicated
- If aneurysm is the underlying cause, surgical intervention may be indicated
- Blood pressure management and control
  - Being aware to not lower blood pressure too quickly or too low

Intracranial Hemorrhage
- Reversal of anticoagulation medications
  - Infusion of fresh frozen plasma (FFP)
  - Vitamin K
  - Protamine sulfate
    - For patients receiving heparin infusions prior to bleeding
- Stop all anticoagulants and antiplatelet medications
- Blood pressure management and control
- ICP monitoring and management
  - Head of bed at 30 degrees
  - Sedation to keep calm
- Medications
  - Mannitol
    - Osmotic therapy
    - Initial dose 0.5 to 1 g/kg
    - Repeat dosing 0.25 to 0.5 g/kg every 4 to 12 hours
    - Dosing should not exceed 250 mg q4h
    - Check serum osmolality
      - Goal 300 mOsmol/kg
  - Hypertonic saline (3%)
    - Osmotic therapy
    - Serum sodium goal 145 to 155 mEq/L
  - Barbiturate coma
    - Pentobarbital is the most used medication
      - Initial bolus 10 to 15 mg/kg
      - 1 to 4 mg/kg/hr maintenance
  - Propofol
    - May help to decrease ICP
  - Hyperventilation

Seizure Management
- Higher risk of seizure in the following:
  - Intracerebral hemorrhage
  - Subcortical hematoma
  - Cortical location
  - Increased risk with the increase in the severity of the stroke
- Medication for prophylaxis based on degree of risk and benefit for patient
- Consider medication in higher-risk patients

Intensive Care Admission Criteria

- Hemodynamic instability
- Airway compromise
- Mechanical ventilation
- Neurological variance
- High risk for bleeding
- Shock
- Ventriculostomy
- Post cardiac arrest
- Continuous antiarrhythmic medication

Complications of Stroke

- Dysphasia
  - Difficulty meeting nutritional needs
  - Increased risk of aspiration
  - May require speech therapy evaluation
- Infection
  - Pneumonia
  - Urinary tract infection
- GI bleeding
  - Patients who develop GI bleeding after CVA have higher mortality
- Incontinence
  - Increase risk for infection
  - Increase risk of skin compromise
- Depression
  - Loss of autonomy
  - May benefit from mental health evaluation once medically stable
- Falls
  - Work with clinical team to prevent falls
  - Falls during hospitalization increase morbidity and mortality
- Delirium
  - Can increase length of stay
  - Can have long-term negative impact on cognitive function

Bibliography

Albers, G. W., Caplan, L. R., Easton, J. D., Fayad, P. B., Mohr, J. P., Saver, J. L., & Sherman, D. G.; TIA Working Group (2002). Transient ischemic attach: Proposal for a new definition. *New England Journal of Medicine, 347*(21), 1713–1716. https://doi.org/10.1056/NEJMsb020987

Chan, L., Hu, C.-J., Fan, Y.-C., Li, F.-Y., Hu, H.-H., Hong, C.-T., & Bai, C.-H. (2018). Incidence of post stroke seizures: A meta-analysis. *Journal of Clinical Neuroscience, 47*(2), 347–351. https://doi.org/10.1016/j.jocn.2017.10.088

Del Zoppo, G. J., Saver, J. L., Jauch, E. C., & Adams, H. P., Jr.; American Heart Association Stroke Council (2009). Expansion of the time window for treatment of acute ischemic stroke with intravenous tissue plasminogen activator: A science advisory from the American Heart Association/American Stroke Association. *Stroke, 40*(8), 2945–2948. https://doi.org/10.1161/STROKEAHA.109.192535

Demaerschalk, B. M., Kleindorfer, D. O., Adeoye, O. M., Demchuk, A. M., Fugate, J. E., Grotta, J. C., Khalessi, A. A., Levy, E. I., Palesch, Y. Y., Prabhakaran, S., Saposnik, G., Saver, J. L., & Smith, E. E.; American Heart Association Stroke Council and Council on Epidemiology and Prevention (2016). Scientific rationale for the inclusion and exclusion criteria for intravenous alteplase in acute ischemic stroke: A statement for healthcare professionals from the American Heart Association/American Stroke Association. *Stroke, 47*(2), 581–641. https://doi.org/10.1161/STR.0000000000000086

Hacke, W., Kaste, M., Bluhmki, E., Brozman, M., Dávalos, A., Guidetti, D., Larrue, V., Lees, K. R., Medeghri, Z., Machnig, T., Schneider, D., von Kummer, R., Wahlgren, N., & Toni, D.; ECASS Investigators (2008). Thrombolysis with alteplase 3 to 4.5 hours after acute ischemic stroke. *New England Journal of Medicine, 359*, 1317–1329. https://doi.org/10.1056/NEJMoa0804656.

McCance, K. L., & Huether, S. E. (2019). *Pathophysiology: The biologic basis for disease in adults children* (8th ed.). Mosby.

Sadaka, F., Jadaw, A., O'Brien, J., & Trottier, S. (2018). Do all stroke patients receiving tPA require ICU admission? *Journal of Clinical Medical Research, 10*(3), 174–177. https://doi.org/10.14740/jocmr3283w

Silverman, I. E., Restrepo, L., & Mathews, G. C. (2002). Poststroke seizures. *Archives of Neurology, 59*(2), 195. https://doi.org/10.1001/archneur.59.2.195

Sorensen, A. G., & Ay, H. (2011). Transient ischemic attack definition, diagnosis, and risk s stratification. *Neuroimaging Clinics of North America, 21*(2), 303–313. https://doi.org/10.1016/j.nic.2011.01.013

ACUTE MANAGEMENT OF SEIZURE ACTIVITY

ACUTE SEIZURES

Causes

- ■ **Epilepsy**
  - ● New onset
  - ● Medication noncompliance
- ■ **Toxins**
  - ● Alcohol withdrawal
  - ● Illicit drug use
  - ● Drug overdose
- ■ **Electrolyte abnormalities**
  - ● Hyponatremia
  - ● Hyperglycemia
  - ● Hypoglycemia
  - ● Hypocalcemia
  - ● Hypomagnesemia
- ■ **Infection**
  - ● Meningitis
  - ● Brain abscess
- ■ **Intracranial process**
  - ● Head trauma
  - ● Acute cerebral vascular accident
  - ● Intracranial bleeding

CLINICAL TIPS AND TRICKS

SEIZURE: WORDS TO KNOW

Status Epilepticus

Status epilepticus: Seizure activity that lasts greater that 30 minutes without cessation or group of seizures that happen in succession without the person regaining full consciousness between seizures.

Post ictal state: State of altered consciousness after seizure. Can last from minutes to hours.

Myoclonus: Irregular jerking movements.

Clonus: Rhythmic jerking movements.

- Central nervous system tumors
- Central venous thrombosis
- **Central nervous system diseases**
  - Alzheimer's disease
  - Central nervous system diseases
  - Vascular disease
- **Other**
  - Sleep deprivation
  - Autoantibodies
  - Eclampsia
  - Stress

Assessment Findings

During seizure
- Neurological
  - Aura
    - Sense prior to seizure
    - Can be visual disturbance or smell
  - Tonic–clonic movements
  - Nystagmus
  - Uncontrolled movements
  - Altered mental status
  - Memory loss
  - Blank stare
  - Posturing
    - Decortication
    - Decerebrating
- Cardiovascular
  - Tachycardia
  - Hypertension
- Respiratory
  - Ictal cry
    - A moan or noise that escapes the pharynx due to contracture of the muscles
  - Cyanosis
  - Apnea
  - Bleeding from mouth or tongue
- Genitourinary
  - Incontinence of bowel or bladder

Post seizure/post ictal phase
- C
  - Altered mental status
    - May last minutes to hours
  - Headache

- Memory loss
- Confusion
- Weakness
- Sleeping
- Cardiovascular
  - Tachycardia
  - Hypotension
- Respiratory
  - Bleeding from mouth or tongue
  - Excessive salivation
- Musculoskeletal
  - Muscle flaccidity
  - Muscle pain

CLINICAL TIPS AND TRICKS

TYPES OF SEIZURES

Typical absence seizures: Sudden brief loss of consciousness. Body control remains intact.

Atypical absence seizures: Sudden loss of consciousness but lasts longer than typical absence seizures.

Generalized tonic–clonic seizures: Starts abruptly without warning and causes tonic muscle contractions.

Atonic seizures: Sudden loss of tone that lasts only seconds.

Myoclonic seizures: Sudden brief muscle contraction that can range from one area of the body to the whole body.

Epileptic seizures: Sustained spasms of flexion and extension.

Diagnostics

Laboratory
- CBC
  - Elevated white blood cell (elevated WBC count)
- Chemistry
  - Hypokalemia
  - Hypocalcemia
  - Hypoglycemia
- Endocrine studies
- Elevated lactic
- Elevated LDH
- Elevated creatinine kinase
- Elevated prolactin level
  - Accurate only if obtained within 30 minutes of seizure activity

- Urinalysis
- Blood alcohol level
- Urine drug screen
- Valproic acid level
  - Check for therapeutic level
  - Therapeutic level 50 to 100 mcg/mL
- Phenytoin level
  - Check for therapeutic level
  - Therapeutic level 10 to 20 mcg/mL

Lumbar puncture
- If infection suspected
- Culture

EEG
- Normal EEG does not rule out seizure activity
- Focal abnormalities—partial seizures
- Generalized abnormalities—primary generalized seizures

Radiology
- Head CT
  - To evaluate acute intracranial pathology
- MRI

CLINICAL TIPS AND TRICKS

KEY SEIZURE MANAGEMENT TIPS
- Airway management is key
  - May need to require oral airway or nasal pharyngeal airway
  - May require intubation for severe anoxia or prolonged or refractory seizure
- Safety
  - Keep from falling
  - Protect from hitting head
- Consider medications when seizure lasts greater than 3 to 5 minutes or for status epilepticus
- Paralytic administration may stop muscle movements but DO NOT stop seizure activity in brain

Treatment and Management

General
- Ensure adequate brain oxygenation.
- Prevent injury and insure safe environment.

Medications
- When to start antiepileptic medications:
  - Patient with any reoccurring seizures
  - Seizure with known cause that is not reversible
  - Single seizure treatment is controversial

■ Antiepileptics in the patient
  ● Keppra
    ■ 500 to 1,000 mg IV bolus
  ● Fosphenytoin sodium
    ■ Prodrug form of phenytoin and is rapidly and completely converted to phenytoin
  ● 10 to 20 mg/kg
■ IV magnesium
  ● Used specifically for eclamptic seizures

Treat underlying cause
■ Underlying cause can often be complicated and require specialty management.
■ Consider neurology consult.

CLINICAL TIPS AND TRICKS

ALCOHOL WITHDRAWAL AND SEIZURE ACTIVITY
■ Goals of alcohol withdrawal management include seizure prevention.
■ Alcohol tolerance can lead to benzodiazepine tolerance and require higher doses.
■ Symptoms preceding seizure include tachycardia, fever, tremors, and/or hallucinations.
■ Benzodiazepines are the most common medication used for alcohol withdrawal prevention.
■ The Clinical Institute Withdrawal Assessment for Alcohol scale, revised (CIWA-AR) score is often used to dose medications to prevent delirium tremens.

STATUS EPILEPTICUS

■ **Definition**
  ● Continuous or repetitive seizures in which patient does not regain wakefulness between events
  ● Emergent situation
  ● Can cause significant neurological injury
■ **Management**
  ● D50 bolus
  ● Thiamine 100 mg IM
  ● Diazepam
    ■ IV ideal dosing
    ■ 0.2 mg/kg
    ■ 20 mg maximum in one dose
  ● Lorazepam
    ■ IV ideal dosing
    ■ 0.1 mg/kg
    ■ 10 mg maximum in one dose
  ● Risk for airway compromise with high dose of benzodiazepines

Bibliography

Beghi, E., Carpio, A., Forsgren, L., Hesdorffer, D. C., Malmgren, K., Sander, J. W., Tomson, T., & Hauser W. A. (2010). Recommendation for a definition of acute symptomatic seizure. *Epilepsia, 51*(4), 671–675. https://doi.org/10.1111/j.1528 -1167.2009.02285.x

Bottaro, F. J., Martinez, O. A., Pardal, M. M., Bruetman, J. E., & Reisin, R. C. (2007). Nonconvulsive status epilepticus in the elderly: A case-control study. *Epilepsia, 48*(5), 966. https://doi.org/10.1111/j.1528-1167.2007.01033.x

Droney, J., & Hall, E. (2008). Status epilepticus in a hospice inpatient setting. *Journal of Pain and Symptom Management, 36*(1), 97–105. https://doi.org/10.1016/ j.jpainsymman.2007.08.009

Huff, J. S., Morris, D. L., Kothari, R. U., & Gibbs, M. A. (2001). Emergency department management of patients with seizures: A multicenter study. *Academic Emergency Medicine, 8*(6), 622–628. https://doi.org/10.1111/j.1553-2712.2001. tb00175.x

Matz, O., Heckelmann, J., Zechbauer, S., Litmathe, J., Brokmann, J. C., Willmes, K., Schulz, J. B., & Dafotakis, M. (2018). Early postictal serum lactate concentrations are superior to serum creatine kinase concentrations in distinguishing generalized tonic-clonic seizures from syncopes. *Internal Emergency Medicine, 13*(5), 749. https://doi.org/10.1007/s11739-017-1745-2

McCance, K. L., & Huether, S. E. (2019). *Pathophysiology: The biologic basis for disease in adults children* (8th ed.). Mosby.

Pellock, J. M. (1998). Management of acute seizure episodes. *Epilepsia, 39* (1), S28–S35.

Walker, M. C. (2003). Status epilepticus on the intensive care unit. *Journal of Neurology, 250*(4), 401. https://doi.org/10.1007/s00415-003-1042-z

SECTION IV
MANAGEMENT OF RENAL AND ELECTROLYTE DISORDERS

8
ACUTE KIDNEY INJURY AND RENAL FAILURE

Prerenal

Causes

- Hypovolemia
  - Volume depletion
    - Hemorrhage
    - Dehydration
    - Diabetes insipidus
  - Decreased circulating volume
    - Hepatorenal syndrome
    - Cirrhosis
    - Congestive heart failure
    - Nephrotic syndrome
- Hypotension
  - Sepsis
  - Shock states
- Renal artery stenosis
- Vasculitis
- Drugs affecting perfusion
  - Cyclosporine
  - Tacrolimus

- Nonsteroidal anti-inflammatory drugs (NSAIDs)
- Angiotensin-converting enzyme (ACE) inhibitors

AZOTEMIA VERSUS UREMIA	
AZOTEMIA	**UREMIA**
• Significantly increases in BUN with or without increase in creatinine • Not associated with specific symptoms • May not be related to kidney injury	• Cluster of symptoms associated with renal failure • Pruritis • Encephalopathy/alterations in mental status • Nausea and/or vomiting

BUN, blood urea nitrogen

Assessment Findings

- Decreased urine output
- Tachycardia
- Shock symptoms
- Altered mental status
- Nausea
- Vomiting

RIFLE AND AKIN CLASSIFICATION		
	RIFLE CRITERIA	**AKIN**
RISK		**STAGE I**
URINE OUTPUT	<0.5 mL/kg/hr	<0.5 mLl/kg/hr For more than 6 hours
CREATININE	>150 from baseline or GFR >25%	>150%–200% from baseline or GFR >25%
INJURY		**STAGE II**
URINE OUTPUT	<0.5 mL/kg/hr	>200%–300% from baseline
CREATININE	>200% from baseline or GFR decreased by >50%	<0.5 mL/kg/hr For more than 12 hours

FAILURE		STAGE III	
URINE OUTPUT	<0.3 mL/kg/hr for more than 12 hours		>300% of baseline or >4 mg/dL with an acute increase of >0.5 mg/dL or on RRT
CREATININE	>300% from baseline or GFR decreased by >75%		Urine output <0.3 mL/kg/hr for more than 12 hours
		LOSS	Complete loss of function for more than 3 months

GFR, glomerular filtration rate; RRT, renal replacement therapy.

Diagnostics

- Laboratory
  - Basic metabolic panel
    - BUN-to-creatinine ratio 20:1
    - Hyperkalemia
  - Complete blood count (CBC)
    - Leukocytosis
- Urinalysis
  - Hyaline casts in urinalysis
  - Decreased urine sodium
  - Increased urine-specific gravity
- Fraction of excreted sodium (FENa)
  - FENa <1%

CLINICAL TIPS AND TRICKS

CALCULATING THE FRACTION OF EXCRETED SODIUM

FENa = (urine sodium/serum sodium)/(urine creatinine/serum creatinine) × 100

Treatment and Management

- Improve hypotension
- Improve perfusion
- Fluid challenge
- Treat underlying condition
- Renal replacement therapy if severe

INTRARENAL

CLINICAL TIPS AND TRICKS

INTRARENAL (INTRINSIC)

■ Intrinsic injuries can be classified by ischemic and nephrotoxic injuries.
■ These are conditions that lead to damage to the functionality of the kidney by damaging part of the structure.
■ Decreased urine output and increase in serum BUN and creatinine after event or exposure.
■ Many different causes with different diagnostics.

ACUTE TUBULAR NECROSIS

Causes

■ Most common intrarenal condition
■ Hypoperfusion causes damage and destruction to the renal tubules
■ Caused by prolonged prerenal conditions

Assessment Findings

■ Current or recent shock state
■ Symptom of volume depletion
■ Decreased urine output
■ Tachycardia
■ Hypotension

Diagnostics

■ BUN/creatinine ratio of 10:1
■ Urine osmolality approximately 300 mOsm/kgH$_2$O
■ Urine sodium > 40 mEq/L
■ FENa >2%
■ Muddy brown casts on urinalysis

Treatment and Management

■ Improve perfusion
■ Avoid hypotension
■ Treat underlying condition
■ Supportive care
■ Acute dialysis may be needed
■ Recovery 1 to 4 weeks

CONTRAST-INDUCED NEPHROPATHY

Causes

- Renal vasoconstriction and direct cytotoxicity of contrast material
  - Patients should be well hydrated with isotonic fluids prior to studies requiring dye injections to decrease risk for contrast-induced nephropathy
  - Benefits of testing should also be considered

Assessment Findings

- Sudden decrease in urine output
- Recent contrast administration
- Edema
- Malaise

Diagnostics

- FeNa <1%
- Serum creatinine increases quickly over 24 to 48 hours after contrast media

Treatment and Management

- Isotonic fluids
- Hemodynamic support; avoid hypotension
- May require renal replacement therapy for electrolyte abnormalities of volume overload

GLOMERULONEPHRITIS

Causes

- Medications
- Immunologic conditions
- Infection
- Vasculitis

Assessment Findings

- Hematuria
- Proteinuria
- Hypertension

■ Edema
■ Bleeding

Diagnostics

■ Laboratory findings
  ● Hyponatremia
  ● Elevated partial thromboplastin time (PTT)
  ● Elevated international normalized ratio (INR)
  ● Low fibrinogen
■ Urinalysis
  ● Blood
  ● Red blood cells
  ● Protein
  ● Dysmorphic erythrocytes
  ● Erythrocyte casts
■ Biopsy

Treatment and Management

■ Supportive treatment recommended in all patients with glomerulonephritis
  ● Blood pressure control
  ● Dialysis
■ Intravenous steroids
  ● Dosing will depend on type

INTERSTITIAL NEPHRITIS

Causes

■ Drug induced
  ● Most common cause
  ● Sulfonamides
  ● Aminoglycosides
  ● Vancomycin
  ● Mannitol
■ Infection
■ Immunological

Assessment Findings

■ Decreased urine output
■ Fever
■ Rash
■ Arthralgias

Diagnostics

- Classic triad (10%–30% of patients)
  - Fever
  - Rash
  - Eosinophilia
  - Mild proteinuria
- BUN-to-creatine ratio variable among patients
- Urine osmolality variable

Treatment and Management

- Discontinue suspected offending medications
- If no improvement of renal function after 5 to 7 days then may warrant further intervention
- Trial of glucocorticoids
  - Treatment of underlying condition

POSTRENAL

CLINICAL TIPS AND TRICKS

POST RENAL

- Urinary obstruction that causes a rise in the renal tubular pressure and eventually decreases the tubular function.
- If obstruction is not removed or urine diverted, permanent damage to the kidney may result.
- If obstruction is bilateral, it can be the cause of permanent renal failure.
- Progressive disease where vascular supply is disrupted and leads to loss of renal function over a period.
- If it goes untreated, permanent renal failure may result.
- Risk increases with advanced age.
- Suprapubic catheter may be indicated in emergent situations where obstruction cannot be bypassed by other methods.

Causes

Renal Calculi

- Types of calculi
  - Hypercalciuric calcium
  - Hyperoxaluric calcium
  - Hyperuricosuria calcium
  - Struvite
  - Uric acid
  - Cystine
  - Hypocitraturia

Assessment Findings

- Renal colic
- Nausea
- Vomiting
- Costovertebral angle tenderness
- Dysuria
- Abdominal or flank pain
- Bladder distention

CLINICAL TIPS AND TRICKS

NEPHROLITHIASIS

- Nephrolithiasis is a condition when stones are in the pelvis, kidney, or ureters.
- These stones are made up of calcium phosphate uric acid, calcium oxalate, struvite, or cystine.
- Some people are more prone to developing stones and may develop many stones over their lifetime.
- There is a higher incidence of stones in men.

Diagnostics and Findings

Laboratory
- CBC
  - Leukocytosis
- Serum uric acid level

Urinalysis
- Blood

Imaging
- CT scan
- Renal ultrasound
- Bladder ultrasound

Treatment and Management

Remove Obstruction
- Irrigate catheter
- Surgical intervention for stone obstructions

Suprapubic Tube in Emergent Situations
- Treat symptoms
  - Pain
  - Nausea and vomiting
- Smaller stones allowed to pass spontaneously
- Larger stones require lithotripsy
- Cystoscopy may be required for large fragment removal
- Long-term management is to prevent reoccurrence
- Antibiotics may be required for concurrent infection

ACUTE CONDITIONS OF THE KIDNEY

CLINICAL TIPS AND TRICKS

RENAL ARTERY STENOSIS

- Progressive disease where vascular supply is disrupted and leads to loss of renal function over a period
- Risk increases with age
- Renal artery stenosis increases risk of coronary artery events such as myocardial infarction
- Decreased blood supply causes ischemia to the kidney
- Reduced blood flow leads to increase in renin, which causes hypertension
- Kidney atrophies from decreased blood flow
- Can lead to chronic renal failure if untreated
- Unaffected kidney will often compensate for a period of time but will eventually fail

RENAL ARTERY STENOSIS

Causes

- Arteriosclerosis of renal arteries
- Fibromuscular dysplasia

Risk Factors

- Advanced age
- Being female
- Underlying hypertension
- Tobacco use
- Diabetes

Assessment Findings

- Sudden onset of hypertension
- Age >50 years
- Resistant hypertension
- Pulmonary edema without history

Diagnostics

- Renal functions
- Serum chemistries
- Urinalysis
- Renal ultrasound

- First-line diagnostic
- May show asymmetric kidneys
- CT angiography
- Invasive angiography
- MRA

Treatment and Management

- Blood pressure control
  - ACE inhibitors
  - ARBS if unable to tolerate ACE
- Statin for atherosclerosis
- Glycemic control
- Smoking cessation
- Restoring blood flow to kidney
  - Stent placement
  - Angioplasty

Bibliography

Chacko, J. (2008). Renal replacement therapy in the intensive care unit. *Indian Journal of Critical Care Medicine, 12*(4), 174–180. https://doi.org/10.4103/0972-5229.45078

Farrar, A. (2018). Acute kidney injury. *Nursing Clinics of North America, 53*(4), 499–510. https://doi.org/10.1016/j.cnur.2018.07.001

Hricik, D. E., Chung-Park, M., & Sedor, J. R. (1998). Glomerulonephritis. *New England Journal of Medicine, 339*(13), 888–899. https://doi.org/10.1056/NEJM199809243391306

Huber, W., Schneider, J., Lahmer, T., Küchle, C., Jungwirth, B., Schmid, R. M., & Schmid, S. (2018). Validation of RIFLE, AKIN, and modified AKIN definition of acute kidney injury in a general ICU. *Medicine, 97*(38), 1–8. https://doi.org/10.1097/MD.0000000000012465

Isaac, S. (2012). Contrast- induced nephropathy: Nursing implications. *Critical Care Nurse, 32*(3), 41–48. https://doi.org/10.4037/ccn2012516

Koyner, J. L. (2012). Assessment and diagnosis of renal dysfunction in the ICU. *Chest, 141*(6), 1584–1594. https://doi.org/10.1378/chest.11-1513

Lao, D., Parasher, P. S., Cho, K. C., & Yeghiazarians, Y. (2011). Atherosclerotic renal artery stenosis- Diagnosis and treatment. *Mayo Clinic Proceedings, 86*(7), 694–657. https://doi.org/10.4065/mcp.2011.0181

McCance, K. L., & Huether, S. E. (2019). *Pathophysiology: The biologic basis for disease in adults children* (8th ed.). Mosby.

Ronco, C., Bellomo, R., & Kellum, J. A. (2019). Acute kidney injury. *Lancet, 394*, 1949–1964. https://doi.org/10.1016/S0140-6736(19)32563-2

Ronco, C., & Ricci, Z. (2008). Renal replacement therapies: Physiological review. *Intensive Care Medicine, 34*, 2139–2146. https://doi.org/10.1007/s00134-008-1258-6

Safian, R. D., & Textor, S. C. (2001). Renal artery stenosis. *New England Journal of Medicine, 344*(6), 431–442. https://doi.org/10.1056/NEJM200102083440607

Vinen, C. S., & Oliveira, D. G. (2002). Acute glomerulonephritis. *Postgraduate Medical Journal, 79*, 206–213. https://doi.org/10.1136/pmj.79.930.206

9

ELECTROLYTE DERANGEMENTS

POTASSIUM

Normal Level
- 3.5 to 5.2 mEq/L

HYPERKALEMIA

CLINICAL TIPS AND TRICKS

POTASSIUM
- Potassium is a vital electrolyte that plays a large part in muscle function.
- Approximately 90% of potassium is intracellular.
- The kidneys are the primary method of excretion.

Causes

- Transcellular shift
  - Rhabdomyolysis
  - Metabolic acidosis
  - Hemolysis
  - Tumor lysis syndrome
  - Hyperglycemia
  - Succinylcholine administration
  - Digoxin toxicity
- Impaired excretion of potassium
  - Acute kidney injury
  - Chronic renal failure
  - Ingestion of potassium foods
  - Potassium supplements
  - Transfusion on blood products
  - Potassium sparing diuretics
  - Sickle cell disease
  - Medications

- Nonsteroidal antiinflammatory drugs
- ACE inhibitors
- ARB
- Bactrim
- Insulin deficiency

CLINICAL TIPS AND TRICKS

HYPERKALEMIA

- Peaked T waves are only seen in a small percentage of patients.
- Chronic hemodialysis patients will often tolerate a high potassium level for a longer period.
- Patient may not have any symptoms.
- Hyperkalemia may be present post cardiac arrest due to hypoperfusion.

Assessment Findings

- Muscle weakness
- Flaccid paralysis
- Cardiac abnormalities
- Symptoms of underlying conditions

Diagnostics

- **Laboratory**
  - Chemistry
    - Serum K level >5.2 mEq/L
  - Serum renin
  - Serum aldosterone
- **EKG**
  - Peaked T waves
  - Prolonged PR intervals
  - Wide QRS
  - V-fib

Treatment and Management

- Limit oral K intake
- Intravenous (IV) hydration
- Furosemide injection IV to increase K excretion
- Sodium polystyrene sulfonate
  - Dose: 25 to 50 g orally or rectally
  - Onset: 1 to 2 hours

Critical-Level Treatment

- **Regular insulin**
  - Dose: 10 units IV

- Onset: 15 minutes
- D50 given to prevent hypoglycemia if patient is euglycemic
- **Calcium**
  - Dose: Calcium gluconate 10% 1G IV
  - Onset: Immediate
- **Albuterol nebulizer**
  - Dose: 10 to 20 mg nebulizer over 15 minutes
  - Onset: 10 to 30 minutes
- **Sodium bicarb**
  - Effective only if there is underlying metabolic acidosis
- **Emergent dialysis treatment in severe cases**

HYPOKALEMIA

Causes

- Decreased intake
- Transcellular shift
  - Insulin excess
  - Beta 2 adrenergic agonist (albuterol)
  - Thyrotoxicosis
- Renal loss
  - Diuretic use
    - Thiazides
    - Loop
    - Acetazolamide
    - Mannitol
- Gastrointestinal (GI) loss
  - Diarrhea
  - Vomiting
  - Nasogastric (NG) suction
- Renal tubular acidosis
- Increased aldosterone
- Renin secreting tumor
- Hypomagnesemia

CLINICAL TIPS AND TRICKS

HYPOKALEMIA
- Most common cause is use of loop diuretics
- Can also be associated with excess water
- In the ICU setting, hyponatremia has been shown to be associated with mortality and a high risk of death

Assessment Findings

- Muscle weakness
- Muscle cramps
- Diaphragm paralysis
- Palpitations
- Flattened T waves on EKG
- Arrhythmias

Diagnostics

- Serum K <3.5 mEq/L
- Lab chemistries
- EKG with flattened T waves
- Low serum Mg level
- Aldosterone
- Renin
- Arterial blood gas (ABG)
  - pH
  - Serum bicarbonate

Treatment and Management

- Supplementation with intravenous potassium
  - Peripheral vein infusion 10 mEq/100 mL
  - Central vein infusion maximum 20 mEq/100 mL
  - Infuse 10 to 20 mEq/hr
  - Patient should be on continuous cardiac monitor during infusion
- Supplementation with oral potassium
  - KCl 10 to 60 mEq
  - May divide dose

Critical-Level Treatment

- Combination of IV and PO (by mouth, if able to tolerate) recommended
- Continuous cardiac monitoring
- Watch for arrhythmias

SODIUM

Normal Level

135 to 145 mEq/L

HYPERNATREMIA

Causes

Hypovolemia/Euvolemia
- Decreased water intake
  - Older adults
  - Nothing by mouth (NPO) due to illness
  - Unable to access free water
  - Impaired thirst
- Insensible water loss
  - Acute burns
  - Large wounds
  - Open abdomen
  - Febrile states
  - Excessive sweating
  - Blistering skin diseases
    - Bullous pemphigoid
    - Toxic epidermal necrolysis
- Osmotic diuresis
  - Water loss
  - Mannitol therapy
- GI loss
  - Excessive diarrhea or emesis
- Surgical drains
- Central diabetes insipidus
- Nephrogenic diabetes insipidus

Hypervolemia
- Hypertonic sodium load
  - Sodium bicarb infusions
  - IV sodium chloride infusion
  - Salt tablets
- Hyperaldosteronism/Cushing's syndrome

Assessment Findings

- Neurologic
  - Stupor
  - Coma
  - Lethargy
  - Confusion
  - Irritability
- GI
  - Nausea
  - Vomiting

- Hypotension
- Tachycardia
- Thirst
- Polyuria
- Symptoms of underlying disease process

Diagnostics

- Serum sodium level greater than 150 mEq/L
- Serum osmolality
- Urine osmolality
- Antidiuretic hormone (ADH) level

Treatment and Management

- Estimate patient's free water deficit (see the following box)
- Replace water at maintenance rate plus deficit
- Aim for reduction of 1 mEq/L every hour
- Frequent electrolyte evaluation
  - At least every 2 to 4 hours
- Oral free water if possible
- IV fluids
  - D5W
    - For mild hypovolemia states
    - Watch for hyperglycemia
  - ½ NS
  - ¼ NS
    - May be beneficial in patients with hyperglycemia who cannot tolerate large volume of D5W
- Treat diabetes insipidus if underlying cause

HYPONATREMIA

Causes

- Thiazide diuretics
- Pseudohyponatremia
  - Sodium corrected for hyperglycemia
- Hypervolemia or excess free water
- Syndrome of inappropriate diuretic hormone (SIADH)
- Cerebral sodium salt wasting

Assessment Findings

- Weakness
- Lethargy

Diagnostics

■ **Laboratory**
  ● Serum chemistry
  ● Serum electrolytes
    ■ Serum sodium level of <135 mEq/L
  ● Serum osmolality
  ● Cortisol
  ● Adrenocorticotropic hormone (ACTH)
■ **Urinalysis**
  ● Urinalysis
  ● Urine electrolytes
  ● Urine osmolality

CLINICAL TIPS AND TRICKS

CALCULATING FREE WATER DEFICIT IN HYPERNATREMIA

Free water deficit (FWD) = Total body water (TBW) × (serum [Na] −140)/140; TBW = weight (kg) × 0.6 (male) or 0.5 (female)

TBW = weight (kg) × 0.6 for males

TBW = weight (kg) × 0.5 for females

If an older adult, use 0.5 for males and 0.45 for females

Treatment and Management

■ Identify and treat underlying cause
■ Normal saline infusion
■ Sodium level should be corrected slowly
■ Electrolytes monitored at regular intervals (q4–8h) while undergoing correction

Critical-Level Treatment

■ Sodium level <120
■ Severe hyponatremia may require hypertonic saline (3%) infusions
■ Electrolytes should be monitored closely (q2–4h)
■ Requires continuous cardiac monitoring

CALCIUM

Normal Level

■ Calcium 8.6 to 10.2 mg/dL
■ Ionized calcium 4.6 to 5.3 mg/dL

CLINICAL TIPS AND TRICKS

CALCIUM

- Most of the body's calcium stored in bone
- Plays a role in muscle and motor function
- Serum calcium can be inaccurate in patients with low albumin

HYPERCALCEMIA

- Increase in total and ionized calcium levels
- With a serum level greater than 10.2 mg/dL or an ionized level greater than 5.3 mg/dL

Causes

- Hyperparathyroidism
  - Most common cause
- Malignancy
  - Especially in lung, renal, or breast cancer
- Vitamin D toxicity
- Granulomatous disease
  - Sarcoidosis
- Vitamin A intoxication
- Hyperthyroidism
- Immobilization or casting
- Thiazide diuretic

Assessment Findings

- Neurologic
  - Lethargy
  - Coma
  - Personality changes
- GI
  - Nausea
  - Vomiting
  - Constipation
- Renal
  - Renal calculi
  - Nocturia
- Musculoskeletal
  - Muscle weakness
  - Bone pain
  - Depressed deep tendon reflexes

- Hypertension
- Confusion
- Weakness

Diagnostics

- **Laboratory**
  - Serum calcium > 10.2 mg/dL
  - Ionized calcium > 5.3 mg/dL
  - Parathyroid hormone (PTH) level
  - Thyroid functions
  - Vitamin D levels
- **EKG**
  - QTc interval

Treatment and Management

- Generally followed unless critical or symptomatic

Severe Acute Hypercalcemia

- IV hydrations
- Calcitonin
- IV biphosphates
  - Pamidronate 90 mg over 24 hours × 7 days
  - Etidronate 7.5 mg/kg over 2 to 3 hours for 3 days
- Diuretics to increase urine output
- Hemodialysis

HYPOCALCEMIA

Causes

- Hypoparathyroidism
  - Seen in patients with thyroidectomy
- Vitamin D deficiency
  - Poor PO intake
  - Severe liver disease
  - P450 enzyme inducers
    - Phenytoin
    - Phenobarbital
    - Isoniazid
    - Rifampin
- Hypomagnesemia
- Uremia
- Hyperphosphatemia
  - Rhabdomyolysis
  - Tumor lysis syndrome

- Pancreatitis
- Alkalemia
- Alcoholism
- Citrate infusion
- Ethylene glycol toxicity

Assessment Findings

- Confusion
- Seizure
- Bradycardia
- Prolong QT interval prolongation
- Bradycardia
- Complete heart block
- Circumoral or distal paresthesia
- Tetany
- Ataxia
- Chvostek's sign
- Trousseau's sign
- Muscle weakness
- Dry skin and nails
  - Seen more in chronic patients

CLINICAL TIPS AND TRICKS

SYMPTOMS OF HYPOCALCEMIA

Trousseau sign: Carpal spasm induced by inflating a blood pressure cuff to upper arm above systolic blood pressure for 3 minutes.

Cvostek sign: Perioral muscle twitching when tapping the ipsilateral facial nerve.

Diagnostics

Laboratory

- Serum calcium level < 8.6 mg/dL
  - Serum calcium should be corrected for hypoalbuminemia
- Ionized calcium level < 4.6 mg/dL
- Albumin
- Magnesium
- Parathyroid hormone (PTH) level
- Thyroid functions
- Vitamin D levels

EKG

- Prolonged QTc interval

Treatment and Management

- *Acute Severe Symptomatic*
  - Calcium chloride 500 mg IV over 5 to 10 minutes
  - Calcium gluconate 2 g IVP
- *Asymptomatic*
  - Calcium carbonate oral 2 to 3 g in divided doses

PHOSPHORUS

Normal Level

2.5 to 4.5 mg/dL

CLINICAL TIPS AND TRICKS

PHOSPHORUS

- Phosphorus is an electrolyte that is important for effective cellular metabolism.
- Most phosphate is intracellular and only a small amount (about 1%) is extracellular.
- Phosphate is regulated by the kidneys, and reabsorption is dependent on vitamin D, insulin, and hormones.
- Parathyroid hormone plays the biggest role in regulation of phosphorus, but calcitonin, thyroid, and growth hormone also have some effect.
- Altered phosphorus levels in ICU are associated with high mortality and morbidity.

HYPERPHOSPHATEMIA

Causes

- Low renal clearance
- Increased tubular phosphorus reabsorption
- Intake from phosphate-based laxatives
- Tumor lysis syndrome
- Acromegaly
- Vitamin D toxicity

CLINICAL TIPS AND TRICKS

HYPOPHOSPHATEMIA

- Hypophosphatemia is common in the ICU but is most often asymptomatic.
- However, suboptimal levels can increase duration of mechanical ventilation and increase risk of ventricular tachycardia.

Assessment Findings

- Grainy feeling to skin
- Pruritis
- Conduction defects
- Acute conjunctivitis

Diagnostics

- Serum phosphorus level > 4.5 mg/dL
- Renal panel or chemistry profile
  - Evaluating for renal insufficiency

Treatment and Management

- Restrict intake
- Dialysis
- Improvement of renal function

Hypophosphatemia

Causes

- Sepsis
- Alcohol withdrawal
- Malnutrition
- Refeeding syndrome
- Ketoacidosis
- Alkalosis
- Hungry bone syndrome
- Trauma
- Surgery

Assessment Findings

- Generally asymptomatic
- Irritability
- Weakness
- Paresthesia

Diagnostics

- Serum phosphorus level < 2.5 mg/dL

Treatment and Management

- Supplementation of phosphorus
  - Oral phosphorus
  - IV phosphorus

MAGNESIUM

Normal Level

1.7 to 2.2 mg/dL

HYPERMAGNESMIA

Causes

- Renal impairment
- Magnesium intake with renal insufficiency
  - Magnesium-based laxatives or bowel prep
  - Antacids
- Large intake of magnesium
  - Treatment of eclampsia
  - Treatment of asthma

Assessment Findings

- Generalized weakness
- Lethargy
- Absent or diminished deep tendon reflexes
- Hypotension
- Nausea and vomiting

Diagnostics

Laboratory
- Serum magnesium level greater than 2.2 mEq/dL
  - Not usually symptomatic until level is greater than 4.0 mEq/dL
- Renal functions

EKG
- Widening of QRS
- Prolonged PR interval
- Possible complete heart block

Treatment and Management

- Stop all magnesium products
- If EKG changes
  - Calcium gluconate IVP 1 to 2 g
  - Hemodialysis

HYPOMAGNESEMIA

Causes

- Renal loss
  - Diuretics
  - Chronic alcohol use
  - Nephrotoxic drugs
    - Aminoglycosides (vancomycin)
    - Amphotericin B
    - Cisplatin
- GI loss
  - Diarrhea
  - Inflammatory bowel disease
- Poor intake
- Diabetic ketoacidosis (DKA)
- Alcohol withdrawal

Assessment Findings

- Muscle weakness
- Tremors
- Seizures
- Trousseau's sign
- Chvostek's sign
- Tremors

Diagnostics

Laboratory

- Serum magnesium level of less than 1.6 mEq/L
- Serum or ionized calcium level
- Potassium

Urinalysis

- Urine magnesium level

EKG

- Prolonged QTc interval
- Ventricular tachycardia
- Ventricular fibrillation

Treatment and Management

- Moderate to severe
  - IV infusion of magnesium sulfate
  - Correct concurrent hypocalcemia

■ Mild
  ● Oral supplementation
    ■ Magnesium chloride
    ■ Magnesium oxide

Bibliography

Adrogue, H. J., & Madias, N. E. (2000). Hypernatremia. *The New England Journal of Medicine, 342*(20), 1493–1499. https://doi.org/10.1056/NEJM200005183422006

Demssie, Y. N., Patel, L., Kumar, M., & Syed, A. A. (2014). Hypomagnesaemia: Clinical relevance and management. *British Journal of Hospital Medicine, 75*(1), 39–43. https://doi.org/10.12968/hmed.2014.75.1.39

Evans, S. K., & Greenberg, A. (2005). Hyperkalemia: A review. *Journal of Intensive Care Medicine, 20*(5), 272–290. https://doi.org/10.1177/0885066605278969

Halperin, M. L., Goldstein, M. B., & Kamel, S. K. (2010). *Fluid, electrolyte, & acid-base balance pathophysiology* (4th ed.). Elsevier.

Kamel, K. S., & Wei, C. (2003). Controversial issues in the treatment of hyperkalemia. *Nephology Dialysis Transplant, 18*, 2215–2218. https://doi.org/10.1093/ndt/gfg323

McCance, K. L., & Huether, S. E. (2019). *Pathophysiology: The biologic basis for disease in adults children* (8th ed.). Mosby.

Noel, J. A., Bota, S. E., Petrcich, W., Garg, A. X., Carrero, J. J., Harel, Z., Tangri, N., Clark, E. G., Komenda, P., & Sood, M. M. (2019). Risk of hospitalization for serious adverse gastrointestinal events associated with sodium polystyrene sulfonate us in patients of advanced age. *JAMA Internal Medicine, 179*(8), 1025–1033. https://doi.org/10.1001/jamainternmed.2019.0631

Rose, B. D., & Post, T. (2005). *Clinical physiology of acid based and electrolyte disorders* (5th ed.). McGraw-Hill.

Wang, A. S., Dhillon, N. K., Linaval, N. T., Rottler, N., Yang, A. R., Margulies, D. R., Ley, E. J., & Barmparas, G. (2019). The impact of IV electrolyte replacement on the fluid balance of critically ill surgical patients. *The American Surgeon, 85*, 1171–1174.

10

MANAGEMENT OF
ACID–BASE BALANCE

ACID–BASE BALANCE AND INTERPRETATION OF ARTERIAL BLOOD GAS

METABOLIC ACIDOSIS

CLINICAL TIPS AND TRICKS

NORMAL ARTERIAL BLOOD GAS VALUES

pH 7.35 to 7.45
$PaCo_2$: 35 to 45 mmHg
PaO_2: 75 to 100 mmHg
HCO_3^-: 22 to 26 mmol/L

Causes

- Elevated Anion Gap
  - Ketoacidosis
    - Diabetic
    - Alcoholic
  - Lactic acidosis
    - Sepsis
    - Hypotension
    - Localized area of hypoperfusion
  - Renal failure
  - Rhabdomyolysis
  - Poisoning
    - Ethylene glycol
    - Methanol
    - Aspirin
- Non-anion Gap
  - Diarrhea
  - Renal tubular acidosis
  - Chronic renal failure

- Adrenal insufficiency
- Acetazolamide therapy

CLINICAL TIPS AND TRICKS

ARTERIAL BLOOD GAS SAMPLING
Allen Test

Blood is occluded at the wrist, and the palm appears white. Ulnar artery is released. If hand color returns to normal, then may proceed with arterial puncture. If flow does not return, then another site should be chosen due to poor collateral circulation.

Assessment Findings

- Specific to underlying cause and degree of acidosis
- C
  - Ill appearing
  - Weakness
  - Lethargy

Respiratory
- Tachypnea
- Increased work of breathing
- Hypoxia

Cardiac
- Tachycardia
- Bradycardia
- New arrhythmia

Diagnostics

Laboratory
- Arterial blood gas
- Serum chemistries
- Lactic
- Alcohol level
  - In suspected alcohol abuse
- Salicylate level
  - If suspected overdose

Treatment and Management

- Treat underlying cause
- General
  - Protect airway
    - May require intubation
- Fluid resuscitation

- Isotonic fluids
  - Sepsis
  - Diabetic ketoacidosis
  - Alcoholic acidosis
  - Poisoning

CLINICAL TIPS AND TRICKS

IMPORTANT FORMULAS FOR ACID–BASE BALANCE
Anion Gap

$Na^+ - (Cl^- + HCO3^-)$ = Anion gap (normal 10–12 mmol/L)

Winter's Formula

Shows degree of respiratory compensation in metabolic acidosis

$PaCo_2 = 1.5 \times HCO_3^- + 8 (\pm 2)$ = Corrected PCO_2

If measured PCO_2 is higher than the result, there is associated respiratory acidosis. If measured PCO_2 is lower, there is respiratory alkalosis.

Calculated Osmolality

$2 \times$ Na + glucose/18 + BUN/2.8 + EtOH/4.6

METABOLIC ALKALOSIS

Causes

- **Low urine chloride (<20)**
  - Vomiting
  - Nasogastric suctioning
  - Diuretic use
  - Severe congestive heart failure (CHF)
- **Normal or high urine chloride (>30)**
  - Primary or secondary hyperaldosteronism
  - Cushing syndrome
  - Licorice ingestion
  - Diuretic use
  - Excess alkali
    - Baking soda ingestion
    - Massive transfusion (citrate)
    - Total peripheral nutrition (acetate)
    - Excess calcium carbonate ingestion

Assessment Findings

- May be asymptomatic
  - Symptoms generally seen with pH > 7.55

■ Delirium
■ Neuromuscular irritability
■ Hypoventilation
■ Hypoxia

Diagnostics

Laboratory

● Arterial blood gas
● Serum chemistries
● Lactic
● Urine chloride

Treatment and Management

■ Low chloride
  ● Chloride administration
    ■ NS
    ■ Potassium chloride
      ● In patients with hypokalemia
■ High chloride
  ● Treatment of underlying condition

RESPIRATORY ACIDOSIS

CLINICAL TIPS AND TRICKS

RESPIRATORY ACIDOSIS

■ As $PaCO_2$ increases, pH decreases
■ $PaCO_2$ rises from hypoventilation
■ Commonly seen in acute and critically ill patients

Causes

■ **Acute respiratory acidosis**
  ● Asthma
  ● Chronic obstructive pulmonary disease (COPD) exacerbation
  ● Oversedation
  ● Narcotic overdose
    ■ Intentional
    ■ Unintentional
  ● Pneumonia
  ● Central nervous system depression
    ■ Guillain-Barré
    ■ Myasthenia gravis
  ● Pneumothorax

■ **Chronic**
  ● COPD
  ● Chronic lung disease
  ● Chronic central nervous system disorders
  ● Pregnancy
  ● High altitude
  ● Obesity

Assessment Findings

Respiratory
■ Anxiety
■ Agitated
■ Apnea

Neurologic
■ Lethargic
■ Obtunded
■ Unresponsive
■ Myoclonic jerking
■ Tremor
■ Papilledema

Diagnostics

Laboratory
■ Arterial blood gas
■ Serum chemistries
■ Lactic

Treatment and Management

■ Treat underlying condition
■ Increase minute ventilation
  ● Increase respiratory rate
  ● Increase tidal volume
■ Respiratory support
  ● Intubation and mechanical ventilation
  ● Bipap
    ■ Only for patient who is spontaneously breathing and can protect airway

CLINICAL TIPS AND TRICKS

CHRONIC RESPIRATORY DISEASE AND CHRONIC ACIDOSIS
■ Patients with chronic respiratory conditions may have chronic compensated respiratory acidosis.
■ In chronic acidosis, it is normal.

(continued)

■ $PaCO_2$ is elevated and usually between 50 and 60 mmHg.
■ HCO^{3-} is elevated for metabolic compensation to chronic respiratory state.
■ Not all COPD patients chronically retain CO_2.
■ Abnormal pH is a sign of an acute condition.

RESPIRATORY ALKALOSIS

CLINICAL TIPS AND TRICKS

RESPIRATORY ALKALOSIS

■ As $PaCO_2$ decreases, pH increases
■ $PaCO_2$ decreases from hyperventilation
■ Less common than respiratory acidosis

Causes

■ Anxiety
■ Pain
■ Sepsis
■ Central nervous system disorders

Assessment Findings

■ Tachypnea
■ Shortness of breath
■ Anxiety
■ Altered/abnormal breathing pattern
  ● Seen with neurological injury

Diagnostics

Laboratory
■ Arterial blood gas
■ Serum chemistries
■ Lactic

Neurological workup
■ For suspected neurological injury

Treatment and Management

■ Medication for anxiety
■ Morphine
  ● Air hunger
■ Treat underlying neurological conditions

BIBLIOGRAPHY

Farrar, A. (2018). Acute kidney injury. *Nursing Clinics of North America, 53*(4), 499–510. https://doi.org/10.1016/j.cnur.2018.07.001

Halperin, M. L., Goldstein, M. B., & Kamel, S. K. (2010) *Fluid, electrolyte, & acid-base balance pathophysiology* (4th ed.). Elsevier.

Koyner, J. L. (2012). Assessment and diagnosis of renal dysfunction in the ICU. *Chest, 141*(6), 1584–1594. https://doi.org/10.1378/chest.11-1513

McCance, K. L., & Huether, S. E. (2019). *Pathophysiology: The biologic basis for disease in adults children* (8th ed.). Mosby.

Rose B. D., & Post, T. (2005). *Clinical physiology of acid-based and electrolyte disorders* (5th ed.). McGraw-Hill.

Wang, A. S., Dhillon, N. K., Linaval, N. T., Rottler, N., Yang, A. R., Margulies, D. R., Ley, E. J., & Barmparas, G. (2019). The impact of IV electrolyte replacement on the fluid balance of critically ill surgical patients. *The American Surgeon, 85*, 1171–1174.

SECTION V

MANAGEMENT
GASTROINTESTINAL DISORDERS

GASTROINTESTINAL BLEEDING

UPPER GASTROINTESTINAL TRACT BLEEDING

Causes

- Peptic ulcer disease

CLINICAL TIPS AND TRICKS

Helicobacter pylori
- Bacteria that infects the lining of the stomach
- Most common cause of peptic ulcer disease
- Testing methods include noninvasive methods
  - Urea breath test
  - Stool antigen
  - Serum testing
- Testing can also be performed by biopsy during endoscopy
- Treated with combination antibiotic therapy and proton pump inhibitor

- Esophageal varices
- Gastritis
- Mallory-Weiss tear

Assessment Findings

CLINICAL TIPS AND TRICKS

HEMORHAGIC SHOCK
- Tachycardia
- Hypotension
- Pallor
- Decreased urine output
- Obvious bleeding

- Signs and symptoms of active bleeding
- Hematemesis
- Melena
- Epigastric pain

Diagnostics

Endoscopy
- Standard of care
- If patient is hemodynamically unstable due to bleeding, endoscopy should be performed within 12 hours of suspected bleed, but ideally as soon as clinically possible.
- C
  - Complete blood count (CBC)
    - Low hemoglobin and hematocrit
  - Chemistry panel
    - Elevated BUN
    - BUN-to-creatinine ratio > 20:1
  - Type and screen
    - Important to have ready if transfusion is needed
- Blood in gastrointestinal (GI) lavage

Treatment and Management

- Fluid resuscitation
  - Crystalloid
  - Colloid
- Transfusion of packed red blood cells (PRBCs)
  - Keep HGB > 7
- Nasogastric tube to suction
- Nothing by mouth (NPO) until bleeding controlled
- Monitoring
  - Frequent hemoglobin and hematocrit checks
  - Close hemodynamic monitoring

UPPER GASTROINTESTINAL TRACT BLEED SPECIAL CONDITIONS

PEPTIC ULCER DISEASE

Causes

- Loss of stomach epithelium that penetrates to the muscularis mucosae
  - Defined as a mucosal break greater than 5 mm
- *H. pylori*
  - Most common cause
- Imbalance between acid and stomach mucosa

- Medications
  - Nonsteroidal anti-inflammatory drugs (NSAIDs)
  - Aspirin
- Alcohol

Assessment Findings

- Epigastric pain
  - Described as gnawing or aching
  - Occurs 1 to 3 hours after eating
  - Relieved by eating or antacids
- Pain on palpation slightly left of midline
- Coffee ground emesis

Diagnostics

- Same as general GI upper bleed

Treatment and Management

- Pantoprazole infusion
  - Recommended for 72 for ulcers with visible bleeding, visible vessel, or adherent clot
- Pantoprazole daily dosing
  - Recommended for ulcers with clean base and no visible bleeding

Esophageal Varices

Causes

- Portal vein hypertension seen in liver disease

Assessment Findings

- Signs of liver failure
  - Ascites
  - Jaundice

Diagnostics

- Same as general GI upper bleed

Treatment and Management

- Endoscopic treatment with banding with rubber bands
- Endoscopic treatment with cyanoacrylate
- If continued bleeding, other measures include the following:
  - Balloon tamponade with Blakemore tube
  - Transjugular intrahepatic portosystemic shunt (TIPSS)

CLINICAL TIPS AND TRICKS

TRANSJUGULAR INRAHEPATIC PORTOSYSTEMIC SHUNT
- For uncontrolled variceal bleeding in patients with cirrhosis
- Performed by radiologist in interventional radiology
- Creates a channel between hepatic vein and branch of portal vein to decrease pressure
- May not be available in all facilities

- Once bleeding controlled, other measures include the following:
  - Vasoconstricting agents such as vasopressin
  - Pantoprazole infusion
  - Antibiotic therapy has been shown to improve outcomes
  - Beta-blocker therapy with propranolol has been shown to decrease rebleed

MALLORY-WEISS TEAR

Causes

- Lacerations of the mucosa at the junction of the esophagus and the proximal stomach
  - Chronic vomiting
  - Heavy alcohol use, especially with vomiting
  - Bulimia
  - Hiatal hernia
  - Blunt abdominal injury
  - Seizures
  - Coughing
  - Advanced age

Assessment Findings

- Pain that radiates to the back
- Non-bloody emesis

Diagnostics

- Same as general GI upper bleed

Treatment and Management

- IV proton pump inhibitor twice per day
- Antiemetics
- Endoscopic intervention
  - Thermal coagulation
  - Hemoclips
  - Band ligation

LOWER GASTROINTESTINAL TRACT

Causes

- **Diverticulosis**
- **Neoplasm**
  - Polyp
  - Carcinoma
- **Vascular**
  - Hemorrhoids
  - Angiodysplasia
  - Post procedure
  - Biopsy
  - Polypectomy
  - Ischemic
  - Radiation induced
- **Inflammatory**
  - Infection
  - Ulcer
  - Inflammatory bowel disease
- **Gastritis**

CLINICAL TIPS AND TRICKS

LOWER GASTROINTESTINAL BLEED

- Less common than upper GI bleed
- Colonic diverticulosis is the most common cause
- Hemorrhoids also common
- Most will present with bright or dark red blood
- Dark tarry stools are usually due to upper GI bleed
- Most lower GI bleeds are self-limiting and will resolve without intervention

Assessment Findings

- Abdominal pain
- Hematochezia
- Nausea
- Vomiting
- Anorexia
- Hypovolemic shock symptoms due to blood loss
  - Hypotension
  - Pallor
  - Tachycardia
  - Altered level of consciousness

Diverticulosis
- Reports of the urge to defecate
- Bloating
- Abdominal cramping

Neoplasm
- Palpable abdominal mass

Diagnostics

Colonoscopy
- Standard initial method of assessment
- Occult or nonemergent bleeding may need additional workup

Laboratory
- CBC
  - Low hemoglobin and hematocrit
- Type and screen

CLINICAL TIPS AND TRICKS

MASSIVE TRANSFUSION OF BLOOD PRODUCTS
- When transfusing PRBC during active bleeding, the patient is losing more than just red blood cells.
- It is recommended that after 4 to 6 units of PRBC in a 24-hour period to consider transfusing other blood components.
- This includes fresh frozen plasma, platelets, and cryoprecipitate.

Treatment and Management

- Dependent on cause of bleeding
- Fluid resuscitation
  - Crystalloid
  - Colloid
- Transfusion of PRBCs
  - Keep HGB >7
- Nasogastric tube to suction
- NPO until bleeding controlled
- Monitoring
  - Frequent hemoglobin and hematocrit checks
  - Close hemodynamic monitoring
- Correction of coagulopathy
  - International normalized ratio (INR) <2.5
  - Plt > 50 × 10/1
- Embolization

Bibliography

Cook, D., & Guyatt, G. (2018). Prophylaxis against upper gastrointestinal bleeding in hospitalized patients. *New England Journal of Medicine, 378*(26), 2506–2516. https://doi.org/10.1056/NEJMra1605507

Gerson, L. B., Fidler, J. L., Cave, D. R., & Leighton, J. A. (2015). ACG clinical guideline: Diagnosis and management of small bowel bleeding. *American Journal of Gastroenterology, 110*, 1265–1287. https://doi.org/10.1038/ajg.2015.246

Laine, L., & Jensen, D. (2012). Management of patients with ulcer bleeding. *American Journal of Gastroenterology, 107*, 345–360. https://doi.org/10.1038/ajg.2011.480

Meehan, C. D., & McKenna, C. G. (2018). Stopping acute upper- GI bleeds: Risk stratification and quick intervention can save lives. *American Nurse Today, 13*(3), 6–8.

Mitra, V., Marrow, B., & Nayar, M. (2012). Management of acute upper gastrointestinal bleeding. *Gastrointestinal Nursing, 10*, 34–39. https://doi.org/10.12968/gasn.2012.10.7.34

Oakland, K., Chadwick, G., East, J. E., Guy, R., Humphries, A., Jairath, V., McPherson, S., Metzner, M., Morris, A. J., Murphy, M. F., Tham, T., Uberoi, R., Veitch, A. M., Wheeler, J., Regan, C., & Hoare, J. (2019). Diagnosis and management of acute lower gastrointestinal bleeding guidelines from the British Society of Gastroenterology. *Gut, 68*, 776–789. https://doi.org/10.1136/gutjnl-2018-317807

Strate, L. L., & Gralnek, I. M. (2016). ACG clinical guideline: Management of patients with acute lower gastrointestinal bleeding. *American Journal of Gastroenterology, 111*, 459–474. https://doi.org/10.1038/ajg.2016.41

12

ACUTE LIVER DYSFUNCTION

LIVER FAILURE

Causes

- Viral hepatitis
  - Hepatitis C most common viral cause
- Cirrhosis
- Alcohol abuse
- Cytomegalovirus
- Drug toxicity
- Toxins
- Metabolic disorders
- Autoimmune disease

Assessment Findings

General
- Weakness
- Fatigue
- Weight loss
- Hypoglycemia

Gastrointestinal
- Anorexia
- Change in bowel habits
- Nausea and vomiting
- Abdominal discomfort
- Diarrhea
- Gastrointestinal (GI) bleed
- Malnutrition

Skin
- Jaundice
- Angiomas
- Pruritis

Cardiovascular
- Edema
- Hypotension

Hematologic
- Anemia
- Coagulopathy
- Thrombocytopenia
  - Not usually less than 50,000
  - Caused by splenic pooling and increased destruction
- Increase in von Willebrand's factor
- Increase D-dimer
- Decreased protein C levels

Neurologic
- Confusion
- Altered mental status
- Cerebral edema

Pulmonary
- Dyspnea
- Hypoxemia

Renal
- Azotemia
- Oliguria
- Hyponatremia
- Hepatorenal syndrome

CLINICAL TIPS AND TRICKS

JAUNDICE LOCATIONS
- Sclera
- Skin
- Urine
- Mucus membranes
- Nail beds
- Tears

Diagnostics

- Laboratory findings
  - Elevated bilirubin
  - Low albumin
  - Coagulopathy
  - Elevated ammonia
  - Elevated transaminases
  - Aspartate transaminase (AST)
  - Alanine transaminase (ALT)
  - Alkaline phosphatase
- Abdominal/pelvis CT scan

- Liver ultrasound
- Liver biopsy
  - Definitive for cirrhosis

CLINICAL TIPS AND TRICKS

LIFE-THREATENING CIRRHOSIS COMPLICATIONS
- Variceal bleeding
- Spontaneous bacterial peritonitis
- Hepatic encephalopathy

Treatment and Management

- Treatment focused on symptom management and preserving remaining function or transplant

Coagulopathy
- Treatment in active bleeding or high-risk bleeding

Hepatic Encephalopathy
- Decrease ammonia level improving encephalopathy
  - Lactulose
  - Neomycin
  - Rifaximin

Hypoglycemia
- Dextrose infusion
  - D5W
  - D10
- Titrate to avoid hypoglycemia

Ascites
- Diuresis
- Spironolactone
- Lasix
- Fluid restriction
- Albumin infusions for fluid shift
- Paracentesis

Portal Hypertension
- Management of symptoms

Pruritis
- Oral antihistamines
- Skin moisturizer

Transplant
- Criteria
  - Model for end-stage liver disease (MELD) score 12 to 15 or develops life-threatening complication of cirrhosis

- No current ETOH or drug use/abuse
- Compliant with medications and appointments
- Good surgical candidate

CLINICAL TIPS AND TRICKS

MODEL FOR END-STAGE LIVER DISEASE SCORE

- Used for age 12 and over
- Three-month survival
- Score range 6 to 40
- Higher the score, higher the mortality
- Value should be no more than 48 hours old
- Exclusions
  - Hepatocellular carcinoma
  - Cystic fibrosis
  - Hepatic artery thrombosis
  - Primary hyperoxaluria

HEPATORENAL SYNDROME

Causes

- Liver failure
- Abnormal vasodilation that leads to central hypovolemia

Symptoms

- Decreased urine output
  - Can be non-oliguric
- Hypotension
- Ascites
- Uremia

Diagnostics

- Renal panel
  - Slow rise in serum creatinine
  - Hyperkalemia
  - Acidosis

Treatment and Management

- Discontinue nephrotoxic drugs
- Stop diuretics
- Albumin infusion for volume

- ▓ Vasoconstrictors
  - ◉ Norepinephrine
  - ◉ Vasopressin
  - ◉ Dopamine
- ▓ Octreotide
- ▓ Midodrine

Bibliography

Acevedo, J. G., & Cramp, M. E. (2017). Hepatorenal syndrome: Update on diagnosis and therapy. *World Journal of Hepatology, 9*(6), 293–299. https://doi.org/10.4254/wjh.v9.i6.293

Erly, B., Carey, W. D., Kapoor, B., McKinney, J. M., Tam, M., & Wang, W. (2015). Hepatorenal syndrome: A review of pathophysiology and current treatment options. *Seminars in Interventional Radiology, 32,* 445–454. https://doi.org/10.1055/s-0035-1564794

European Association for the Study of the Live. (2010). EASL clinical practice guidelines on the management of ascites, spontaneous bacterial peritonitis, and hepatorenal syndrome in cirrhosis. *Journal of Hepatology, 53,* 397–417.

Francoz, C., Durand, F., Kahn, J. A., Genyk, Y. S., & Nadim, M. K. (2019). Hepatorenal syndrome. *Clinical Journal of the American Society of Nephrology, 14,* 774–781. https://doi.org/10.2215/CJN.12451018

Herrera, J. L., & Rodriguez, R. (2006). Medical care of the patient with compensated cirrhosis. *Gastroenterology & Hepatology, 2*(2), 124–133.

Kamath, P. S., & Kim, R. (2007). The model for end-stage liver disease (MELD). *American Association for the Study of Liver Diseases, 45*(3), 797–805. https://doi.org/10.1002/hep.21563

McCance, K. L., & Huether, S. E. (2019). *Pathophysiology: The biologic basis for disease in adults children* (8th ed.). Mosby.

Peck-Radiosavljevic, M., Angeli, P., Cordoba, J., Farges, O., & Valla, D. (2015). Managing complications in cirrhotic patients. *United European Gastroenterology Journal, 3*(1), 80–94. https://doi.org/10.1177/2050640614560452

13

ACUTE DYSFUNCTION OF THE PANCREAS AND BILIARY SYSTEM

ACUTE PANCREATITIS

PANCREATITIS CLASSIFICATION

Mild Acute Pancreatitis

■ No organ failure or systemic complications

Moderately Severe Acute Pancreatitis

■ Organ failure that is no sustained or local complications; all organ failure resolves

Severe Acute Pancreatitis

■ One or more organ system failure

Causes

■ Stone in biliary tract
■ Alcohol abuse
■ Medications
  ● Azathioprine (Imuran)
  ● Sulfonamides
  ● Furosemide
  ● Valproic acid
■ Post endoscopic retrograde cholangiopancreatography (ERCP)
■ Uncontrolled hyperlipidemia
■ Abdominal trauma
■ Ischemia

Assessment Findings

■ Symptoms occurred suddenly
■ Sudden onset of epigastric or right upper quadrant pain
  ● Pain is usually described as constant and severe
  ● May radiate to back
  ● Is worse with movement
■ Nausea

- Vomiting
- Diaphoresis
- Dyspnea
- Epigastric tenderness
- Fever
- Tachycardia
- Hypotension
- Jaundice
- Cullen's sign
- Grey Turner sign

CLINICAL TIPS AND TRICKS

SIGNS OF PANCREATITIS

- **Cullen's sign**
  - Ecchymosis of the periumbilical region
  - Can be a sign of pancreatic necrosis
- **Grey Turner's Sign**
  - Ecchymosis to the flank
  - Can be a sign of retroperitoneal bleeding

CLINICAL TIPS AND TRICKS

APACHE II SCORE

Developed for use in the ICU to evaluate the severity of pancreatitis

- Age
- Glasgow Coma Scale
- Mean arterial pressure
- FiO_2
- PaO_2
- pH
- Serum sodium
- Serum potassium
- Hct
- White blood cell (WBC)
- Chronic disease

Diagnostics

Laboratory

- Elevated serum amylase
  - Usually 3× the upper limit of normal
  - Elevation within 6 to 12 hours

- Elevate serum lipase
  - Elevated in 4 to 6 hours
  - Peaks at 24 hours
- Leukocytosis
- Bilirubin may be elevated

Radiologic

- Abdominal x-ray (KUB)
  - Ileus may be present
- Abdomen CT with contrast if possible
  - Evaluation of fluid collection

Treatment and Management

- Absolutely nothing by mouth (NPO) initially
- Pain control
  - May require multimodality pain control
- Intravenous (IV) fluids to replace and maintain intravascular volume
  - Crystalloid solution
  - 5 to 10 mL/kg/hr
- Nasogastric tube to suction for ileus or uncontrolled vomiting
- Hourly glucose monitoring
- Insulin for hyperglycemia
- Electrolyte monitoring and replacement
- I&O monitoring hourly
- Bladder pressure monitoring
  - Evaluate for possible abdominal compartment syndrome

ACUTE CHOLECYSTITIS

Causes

- Gall stones
  - Stones lodge in cystic duct
  - Inflammation due to blockage
- Acalculous cholecystitis
  - Seen in critically ill patients
  - Increases mortality
- Ischemia
- Infection
- Tumor
- Stricture of the bile duct

CLINICAL TIPS AND TRICKS

MURPHY SIGN
Murphy sign

Examiner places hand over the right subcostal area (right upper quadrant) and has patient take a deep breath. If patient has pain on inspiration, the sign is positive.

Pain occurs when gallbladder comes in contact with provider's hand.

Sonographic Murphy sign
Pain on inspiration while ultrasound probe is visualizing the gallbladder.

Assessment Findings

- Biliary colic
  - Sudden severe pain to the right upper quadrant
  - May radiate to shoulder or back
- Nausea
- Vomiting
- Anorexia
- Fever
- Murphy's sign
- Jaundice
- May have several episodes before patient seeks care

CLINICAL TIPS AND TRICKS

RANSON'S CRITERIA
Hour zero (each worth 1 point)

- Age >55 years
- WBC >16,000 mcL
- Glucose >200 mg/dL
- Lactate dehydrogenase (LDH) >350 IU/L
- Aspartate transaminase (AST) >250 IU/L

48 hours (each worth 1 point)

- Hct drop of 10% or more
- BUN increase by 5 mg/dL
- Serum calcium <8 mg/dL
- PaO_2 <60 mmHg
- Base deficit >4 mEq/L
- Fluid sequestration >6,000 mL

Results

0 to 2 points: Mortality 0% to 3%
3 to 5 points: Mortality 11% to 15%
6 to 11 points: Mortality >40%

Diagnostics

■ Right upper quadrant ultrasound
  ● Best study for diagnosing gallstones
■ Leukocytosis
■ Elevated serum bilirubin
■ Elevated alanine transaminase (ALT)
■ Elevated AST
■ Elevated LDH
■ Elevated alkaline phosphatase
■ Elevated amylase
■ HIDA scan

Treatment and Management

■ NPO initially
■ Then patient may be able to be slowly advanced to low-fat meals
■ IV fluids for hydration
■ Pain control
■ General surgery evaluation for cholecystectomy
■ Percutaneous drain for acalculous cholecystitis

Bibliography

Banks, P. A. (1997). Practice guidelines in acute pancreatitis. *The American Journal of Gastroenterology, 92*(3), 377–396. https://doi.org/10.1111/j.1572-0241.2006.00856.x

Banks, P. A., & Freeman, M. L. (2006). Practice guidelines in acute pancreatitis. *The American Journal of Gastroenterology, 101*(10), 2379–2400. https://doi.org/10.1111/j.1572-0241.2006.00856.x

Ganpathi, I. S., Diddapur, R. K., Euguene, H., & Karim, M. (2007). Acute acalculous cholecystitis: Challenging the myths. *HPB, 9*, 131–134. https://doi.org/10.1080/13651820701315307

Indar, A. A., & Beckinham, I. J. (2002). Acute cholecystitis. *British Medical Journal, 325*, 639–643. https://doi.org/10.1136/bmj.325.7365.639

McCance, K. L., & Huether, S. E. (2019). *Pathophysiology: The biologic basis for disease in adults children* (8th ed.). Mosby.

Pandol, S. J., Saluja, A. K., Imrie, C. W., & Banks, P. A. (2007). Acute pancreatitis: Bench to bedside. *Gastroenterology, 132*(3), 1127–1151. https://doi.org/10.1053/j.gastro.2007.01.055

Swaroop, V. S., Chari, S. T., & Clain, J. E. (2004). Severe acute pancreatitis. *JAMA, 291*(23), 2865–2868. https://doi.org/10.1001/jama.291.23.2865

Trowbridge, R. L., Rutkowski, N. K., & Shojania, K. G. (2003). Does this patient have acute cholecystitis. *JAMA, 289*(1), 80–86. https://doi.org/10.1001/jama.289.1.80

Whitcomb, D. C. (2006). Acute pancreatitis. *New England Journal of Medicine, 354*(20), 2142–2150. https://doi.org/10.1056/NEJMcp054958

14

MANAGEMENT OF ACUTE INFLAMMATORY GASTROINTESTINAL DISORDERS

DIVERTICULITIS

Types

- Uncomplicated
- Complicated
  - Considered complicated if one or more is present
    - Abscess formation
    - Peritonitis
    - Obstruction
    - Fistula
    - Sepsis
    - No improvement with medical management

CLINICAL TIPS AND TRICKS

DIVERTICULITIS: ADMISSION CRITERIA

- Signs of sepsis
- Inability to take oral
- Fever >102 °F
- Leukocytosis >12 × 10^9/L
- Age >70 years
- Failed outpatient treatment
- Multiple comorbidities
- Immunosuppression
- Perforation or microperforation
- Poorly controlled abdominal pain

Causes

- Inflammation or perforation of diverticulum
- Abscess formation within a diverticulum
- Diverticulum occurs for a variety of reasons
  - Low fiber diet

■ Some research shows that this may not have as much impact as previously thought.
- Decreased bowel motility
- Weakness in the colon wall
- Deranged microbiome
- Diet high in red meat
- Smoking
- Obesity
- Physical inactivity
- Nuts, corn, seeds are no longer considered risk factors

Assessment Findings

■ Abdominal pain
- Pain is acute or subacute
- Left quadrant in most patients
- Suprapubic pain
- Tenderness on palpation
- Guarding
- Pain worse with movement
■ Fever
■ Nausea without vomiting
■ Reports change in bowel habits
■ Constipation alternating with diarrhea
■ Hypoactive bowel sounds on auscultation
■ Urinary symptoms from inflamed colon near bladder
- Dysuria
- Urgency
- Frequency
■ Abdominal distention may indicate bowel obstruction
■ May have symptoms of sepsis or septic shock

Diagnostics

Laboratory
■ Complete blood count (CBC)
- Leukocytosis
■ C-reactive protein
- Elevated

Imaging
■ CT scan with oral and IV contrast if appropriate
- Showing abscess form
■ Abdominal ultrasound
■ Abdominal x-ray (KUB)
- Not diagnostic for diverticulitis
- Will be useful in diagnosis of pneumoperitoneum in perforation
- Diagnostic for bowel obstruction

CLINICAL TIPS AND TRICKS

DIVERTICULUM PERFORATION

Microperforation: Small amounts of gas or air bubbles seen on CT. No obvious free air or free contrast media.

Perforation: Noted free air on CT with possible fluid or contrast spillage. Will lead to peritonitis.

Treatment and Management

- Based on severity
  - Uncomplicated
    - Bowel rest
      - NPO 24 to 48
      - Clear liquids
    - Antibiotic therapy
  - Complicated
    - NPO
      - Nasogastric tube for stomach decompression
    - Intravenous fluids
      - Crystalloid
      - May need increased fluid if vomiting or diarrhea is present
    - Antibiotics
      - Anaerobic coverage
        - Metronidazole
      - Gram-negative coverage
        - Aminoglycoside
        - Third-generation cephalosporin
        - Betalactam
    - Pain management
      - Nonsteroidal anti-inflammatory drugs (NSAIDs) can increase perforation; avoid
      - Acetaminophen
      - Dicyclomine and other antispasmodics
      - Narcotics may be required in complicated and severe cases but can also increase risk of perforation
        - Morphine is the narcotic of choice.

CLINICAL TIPS AND TRICKS

CRITERIA FOR DISCHARGE

- Vital signs return to baseline
- Normalized white blood cell (WBC) count
- Tolerance of oral diet
- Resolution of abdominal pain

- Surgical consult
  - Indications
    - Abscess
    - Peritonitis
    - Patient not improving with medical management

APPENDICITIS

Causes

- Acute inflammation of the vermiform appendix
- Luminal obstruction with a fecalith
  - Can lead to perforation and gangrene
- Inflammation
- Tumors
- Strictures
- Alterations in the colonic microbiome

Assessment Findings

- Abdominal pain
  - Initially central abdomen
  - Migrates right lower quadrant pain
    - Guarding
    - Tenderness on palpation
  - Rovsing's sign
  - Psoas sign
  - Obturator sign
  - Flexion of thigh lessens pain
  - Movement usually worsens pain

CLINICAL TIPS AND TRICKS

SIGNS OF APPENDICITIS

- Rovsing's sign
  - Right lower quadrant pain when pressure applied to left lower quadrant
- Psoas sign
  - Pain with extension of right thigh
- Obturator sign
  - Pain with internal rotation of flexed right thigh

- Anorexia
- Nausea without vomiting
- Urge to defecate
- Low-grade fever

Diagnostics

Laboratory
- CBC
  - Leukocytosis
  - Usually 10,000 to 20,000/mcL
- Urinalysis
  - Elevated specific gravity
  - Hematuria
  - Pyuria

Ultrasound
- Accurate when appendix can be visualized
- Generally used as first approach when perforation not suspected

CT scan
- Used to identify perforation or possible abscess

Treatment and Management

- Antibiotics
  - May be considered before surgical intervention in mild or uncomplicated cases
  - Criteria
    - Adult
    - Not pregnant
    - No evidence of abscess
    - No perforation
    - No suspicion of sepsis
    - Patient will be assessed q6 to 12h for changes in condition
- Surgical consultation
  - Appendectomy
    - Most performed laparoscopy
    - Open
  - Not all appendicitis requires surgical intervention
- Intravenous fluids
- Pain management
  - IV pain medication for pain control

PERITONITIS

Causes

- Primary
  - Spontaneous bacterial peritonitis in patients with cirrhosis
  - *Escherichia coli* most common cause
- Secondary
  - Peritoneal dialysis

- Abdominal trauma
- Penetrating abdominal wounds
- Colon perforation
- Postoperative

CLINICAL TIPS AND TRICKS

PERITONEAL DIALYSIS
- Usually caused by skin bacteria
  - Staphylococcus epidermidis
  - Staphylococcus aureus
- Translocation
  - From gastrointestinal (GI) source

Assessment Findings

- Abdominal pain
  - Worse with motion
  - Rebound tenderness
  - Rigidity
- Abdominal distention
  - Possible ascites
- Decreased bowel sounds
- High fever
- Nausea
- Vomiting
- Constipation
- Tachypnea
- Dyspnea

Diagnostics

Laboratory
- CBC
  - Leukocytosis
  - Elevated hematocrit
- Renal panel
  - Elevated BUN
- Elevated amylase

Peritoneal aspirate
- Elevated WBC
- Elevated LDH
- Protein level elevated
- Glucose less than 50 mg/dL
- Bacteria on gram stain

Blood cultures
- Positive in approximately 25% of patients

Imaging
- Chest x-ray
  - Elevated diaphragm
- CT scan
  - Intra-abdominal mass

Treatment and Management

- Surgical consultation
- Antibiotic therapy
  - Gram-positive and gram-negative coverage until source identified
  - Third-generation cephalosporin
- Fluid resuscitation
  - Crystalloid for fluid replacement
  - Maintenance fluids while NPO to avoid volume deficit
- NPO
  - Nasogastric tube to wall suction
- Respiratory support
- Peritoneal dialysis
  - Antibiotics often instilled into peritoneal catheter
  - Patients may require hemodialysis during acute treatment phase

CLINICAL TIPS AND TRICKS

SPONTANEOUS BACTERIAL PERITONITIS IN CIRRHOSIS

- Patients with cirrhosis and ascites are at high risk for spontaneous bacterial peritonitis
- Usually due to gut bacteria
  - E. coli
  - Klebsiella
- Broad-spectrum antibiotics recommended
  - Third-generation cephalosporin
- Patients with ascites and suspected infection should have diagnostic paracentesis to rule out spontaneous bacterial peritonitis

Bibliography

Flum, D. R. (2015). Acute appendicitis: Appendectomy or the "antibiotic first" strategy. *New England Journal of Medicine, 372*(20), 1937–1943. https://doi.org/10.1056/NEJMcp1215006

MacIntosh, T. (2018). Emergency management of spontaneous bacterial peritonitis: A clinical review. *Cureus, 10*(3), e2253. https://doi.org/10.7759/cureus.2253

Morris, A. M., Regenbogen, S. E., Hardiman, K. M., & Hendren, S. (2014). Sigmoid diverticulitis: A systematic review. *JAMA, 311*(3), 287–297. https://doi.org/10.1001/jama.2013.282025

Siletz, A., Grotts, J., Lewis, C., Tillou, A., Cheaito, A., & Cryer, H. (2018). Monitoring complications of medically managed acute appendicitis. *The American Surgeon, 84,* 1684–1690.

Soares-Weiser, K., Paul, M., Brezis, M., & Leibovici, L. (2002). Antibiotic treatment for spontaneous bacterial peritonitis. *BMJ, 324,* 100–102. https://doi.org/10.1136/bmj.324.7329.100

Such, J, & Runyon, B. A. (1998). Spontaneous bacterial peritonitis. *Clinical Infectious Disease, 27,* 669–676. https://doi.org/10.1086/514940

Swanson, S. M., & Strate, L. L. (2018). In the clinic: Acute colonic diverticulitis. *Annals of Internal Medicine, 168*(9), ITC65–ITC80. https://doi.org/10.7326/AITC201805010

SECTION VI
MANAGEMENT OF ENDOCRINE DISORDERS

ACUTE MANAGEMENT OF DIABETIC EMERGENCIES

DIABETIC KETOACIDOSIS

Causes

- New-onset type I diabetes
- Infection
- Noncompliance
  - Lack of insulin
  - Poor regulation of food intake
- Pancreatitis
- Surgical intervention
- Trauma
- Medications that alter the metabolization of carbohydrates
  - Glucocorticoids
- Cocaine use

CLINICAL TIPS AND TRICKS

HYPERGLYCEMIA OF THE CRITICALLY ILL

- Caused by stress response in the critically ill
- Target glucose between 140 and 180 mg/dL
- Hyperglycemia associated with poor outcomes in critically ill patients
- Critically ill patients should have routine glucose monitoring
- Sliding scale helpful in glucose control

Assessment Findings

General

- Flushed dry skin
- Weight loss
- Weakness
- Fruity breath
- Hypothermia
- Dry mucous membranes

Cardiovascular
- Tachycardia
- Hypotension
- Orthostatic hypotension

Neuro
- Headache
- Encephalopathy
- Coma

Gastrointestinal
- Nausea
- Vomiting
- Abdominal pain

Pulmonary
- Tachypnea
- Kussmaul respiration

Renal
- Polyuria
- Polydipsia

CLINICAL TIPS AND TRICKS

COMPLICATIONS OF DIABETES
- Diabetic retinopathy
- Cardiovascular disease
- Cataracts
- Glaucoma
- Neuropathy
- Increased risk for infections
  - Vaginal and oral yeast infections
- Foot wounds

Diagnostics

Laboratory
- Chemistries
  - Serum glucose greater than 250 mg/dL
    - Usually between 350 and 500 mg/dL
    - Not usually >800 mg/dL
  - Hyperkalemia
    - Due fluid loss
  - Anion gap
  - Increased BUN
  - Hyponatremia
  - Normal serum osmolality

- Serum ketones
- Hemoglobin A1c
- Complete blood count (CBC)
  - Leukocytosis
  - Elevated hematocrit
- Arterial blood gas
  - Arterial pH less than 7.3
- Urinalysis
  - Ketones in serum and urine
  - Glucose in urine

EKG

Treatment and Management

- Close hemodynamic monitoring
- Fluid resuscitation
  - Should be the first intervention, especially in patients with dehydration
  - Bolus of NS 1,000 mL over first hours
  - Isotonic fluids
    - Normal saline 5 to 20 mL/kg/hr
      - Use ideal body weight
    - When glucose is between 200 and 250 mg/dL fluids should be changed to fluids containing dextrose
- Electrolyte replacement
  - Follow potassium closely during acute phase
  - Insulin should be held if potassium less than 3.3
- Insulin therapy
  - Regular insulin per the standard
  - Fast-acting insulin used in some places
  - Long acting not used during acute phase of management
  - Bolus initially
    - Should be given IV
    - Continuous insulin infusion
  - IV insulin should be continued until anion gap is resolved
  - Mild diabetic ketoacidosis (DKA) may be treated with subcutaneous insulin but still requires close monitoring

HYPERGLYCEMIC HYPEROSMOLAR STATE

Causes

- New type II diabetes
- Infection
- Noncompliance
  - Omission of medications
  - Poor regulation of food intake

- Surgical intervention
- Trauma
- Medications that alter the metabolization of carbohydrates
  - Glucocorticoids

Assessment Findings

General
- Flushed dry skin
- Weight loss
- Weakness
- Hypothermia
- Dry mucus membranes

Cardiovascular
- Tachycardia
- Hypotension
- Orthostatic hypotension

Neuro
- Headache
- Encephalopathy
- Coma

Gastrointestinal
- Nausea
- Vomiting
- Abdominal pain

Pulmonary
- Tachypnea

Renal
- Polyuria
- Polydipsia

Diagnostics

Laboratory
- Chemistries
  - Serum glucose greater than 500 mg/dL
    - Usually >1,000 mg/dL
  - Hyperkalemia
    - Due fluid loss
  - No anion gap
  - Increased BUN
  - Increased creatinine
  - Hyponatremia
  - Elevated serum osmolality
- Hemoglobin A1c

■ CBC
  ● Leukocytosis
  ● Elevated hematocrit
■ Arterial blood gas
  ● Arterial pH less than 7.3
■ Urinalysis
  ● In serum and urine
  ● Glucose in urine
    ■ Not always good indicator in type 2 diabetes; many oral medications increase glucose excretion in urine

EKG

CLINICAL TIPS AND TRICKS

SOMOGYI EFFECT AND DAWN PHENOMENON
SYMOGYI EFFECT

■ Nocturnal hypoglycemia develops in the middle of the night, which causes the rise of blood sugar and elevated morning glucose.
■ Treated by decreasing or eliminating bedtime dose of insulin.

DAWN PHENOMENON

■ Decreased sensitivity to insulin due to growth hormone. This causes a progressive rise in glucose overnight, resulting in elevated glucose in the morning.

Treatment and Management

■ Close hemodynamic monitoring
■ Fluid resuscitation
  ● Should be the first intervention, especially in patients with dehydration
  ● Bolus of NS 1,000 mL over the first hour
  ● Isotonic fluids
    ■ Normal saline 5 to 20 mL/kg/hr pending volume status
      ● Use ideal body weight
    ■ When glucose is between 200 and 250 mg/dL, fluids should be changed to fluids containing dextrose
■ Electrolyte replacement
  ● Follow potassium closely during acute phase
  ● Insulin should be held until potassium can be corrected if potassium is less than 3.3
■ Insulin therapy
  ● Regular insulin per the standard
  ● Fast-acting insulin used in some places
  ● Long acting not used during acute phase of management

- Bolus initially
  - Should be given IV
  - Continuous insulin infusion
- IV insulin should be continued until anion gap is resolved

CLINICAL TIPS AND TRICKS

HYPERGLYCEMIA

- Fluid resuscitation is priority in both DKA and hyperglycemic hyperosmolar state (HHS) and should be initial method of treatment.
- Insulin infusion is usually required for gradual glycemic control.
- As serum glucose is lowered, serum potassium level decreases. Frequent potassium monitoring and replacement are often required in both DKA and HHS.

Bibliography

Filers, E., Bianco, A. C., Langouche, L., & Boelen, A. (2015). Endocrine and metabolic considerations in critically ill patients. *Lancet Diabetes Endocrinology, 3*(10), 816–825. https://doi.org/10.1016/S2213-8587(15)00225-9

Finfer, S., Chittock, D., Li, Y., Foster, D., Dhingra, V., Bellomo, R., Cook, D., Dodek, P., Hebert, P., Henderson, W., Heyland, D., Higgins, A., McArthur, C., Mitchell, I., Myburgh, J., Robinson, B., & Ronco, J. (2009). Intensive versus conventional glucose control in critically ill patients. *New England Journal of Medicine, 360*(13), 1283–1297. https://doi.org/10.1007/s00134-015-3757-6

Finney, S. J., Zekveld, C., Elia, A., & Evans, T. W. (2003). Glucose control and mortality in critically ill patients. *JAMA, 290*(15), 2041–2047. https://doi.org/10.1001/jama.290.15.2041a

French, E. K., Donihi, A., & Korytkowski, M. T. (2019). Diabetic ketoacidosis and hyperosmolar hyperglycemic syndrome: Review of acute decompensated diabetes in adult patients. *BMJ, 365*, 1–15. https://doi.org/10.1136/bmj.l1114

Gillespie, G. L., & Campbell, M. (2002). Diabetic ketoacidosis. *AJN, 102*, 13–16.

Johnston, J. A., & Van Horn, E. R. (2011). The effects of correction insulin and basal insulin on inpatient glycemic control. *Medsurg Nursing, 20*(4), 187–193.

Kitabchi, A. E., Umpierrez, G. E., Miles, J. M., & Fisher, J. N. (2009). Hyperglycemic crises in adult patients with diabetes. *Diabetes Care, 32*(7), 1335. https://doi.org/10.2337/dc09-9032

Kraut, J. A., & Madias, N. E. (2012). Treatment of acute metabolic acidosis: A pathophysiologic approach. *Nature Reviews: Nephrology, 8*(10), 589–601. https://doi.org/10.1038/nrneph.2012.186

McCance, K. L., & Huether, S. E. (2019). *Pathophysiology: The biologic basis for disease in adults children* (8th ed.). Mosby.

Van Den Berghe, G., Wouters, P., Weekers, F., Verwaest, C., Bruyninckx, F., Schetz, M., Vlasselaers, D., Ferdinande, P., Lauwers, P., & Bouillon, R. (2001). Intensive insulin therapy in critically ill patients. *New Journal of Medicine, 345*(19), 1359–1367. https://doi.org/10.1056/NEJMoa011300

16

THYROID EMERGENCIES

MYXEDEMA COMA

Causes

Underlying preexisting hypothyroidism and one of the following:

- Infection
- Sepsis
- Myocardial infarction
- Congestive heart failure
- Cold exposure
- Postoperative
- Sedation
- Illicit drug use
  - Opiates
  - Marijuana

Amiodarone
- With or without preexisting hypothyroidism

CLINICAL TIPS AND TRICKS

MYXEDEMA COMA

- Medical emergency
- High mortality
- Patient requires ICU admission
- Occurs more often in winter months
- Not usually seen as the initial presentation of undiagnosed hypothyroidism
- Causes global decrease in organ function
- Can be secondary to noncompliance with medication use

Assessment Findings

Neurological
- Decreased level of conscious
- Altered mental status
- Confusion

Hemodynamics
- Hypotension
- Hypothermia
- Bradycardia
- Low respiratory rate
- Decreased cardiac output

General
- Non-pitting edema
  - Face
  - Tongue
  - Lips
  - Hands
  - Nose

Gastrointestinal
- Abdominal distention
- Hypoactive or absent bowel sounds
- Constipation

Musculoskeletal
- Muscle weakness
- Woltman's sign
  - Delayed relaxation of deep tendon reflexes

Diagnostics

Laboratory
- Chemistry
  - Hypocalcemia
  - Hyponatremia
  - Hypoglycemia
- Thyroid functions
  - High thyroid stimulating hormone (TSH)
    - In primary hypothyroidism
  - Low or normal TSH
    - In central hypothyroidism
  - Low T3
  - Low T4
- Complete blood count (CBC)
  - Anemia
  - Thrombocytopenia
- Cortisol
  - May be low if concurrent adrenal insufficiency
- Coagulation
  - Elevated partial thromboplastin time (PTT)
  - Elevated international normalized ratio (INR)
  - Decreased fibrinogen

■ Arterial blood gas
  ● Elevated PCO_2
  ● Acidosis

Microbiology
■ Blood cultures
  ● If infection suspected as underlying cause
■ Urine culture
  ● If infection suspected

Radiography
■ Chest x-ray
  ● Pleural effusion
■ Kidney, ureter, and bladder (KUB)
  ● Ileus
  ● Constipation

ECHO
■ Pericardial effusion

Treatment and Management

Medications
■ T4
  ● Initial dose 200 to 400 mcg IV × 1 dose
  ● Then 50 to 100 mcg IV daily
    ■ Continue until able to take PO dosing
■ T3
  ● Initial dose 5 to 20 mcg IV × 1 dose
  ● Then 2.5 to 10 mcg q8h
■ T3 and T4 levels should be monitored q24 to 48h
  ● Dosage should be adjusted based on levels

Hemodynamic Support
■ Vasopressors may be required for blood pressure support until underlying condition can be corrected
■ Dopamine
  ● May treat both bradycardia and hypotension
■ Norepinephrine
■ Epinephrine

Respiratory
■ Consider intubation for the following:
  ● Hypoventilation
  ● Airway protection for altered consciousness
■ Follow arterial blood gas (ABG) for ventilatory status
■ Follow chest x-ray 24 to 48 hours
■ Pleural effusions will generally resolve without intervention when myxedema resolves

Hypothermia
- Aggressive warming measures not indicated due to risk of vasodilation and increased hypotension
- Warm room
- Apply room temperature blankets

Hypoglycemia
- Frequent blood glucose monitoring
- May require dextrose boluses and infusion

ADRENAL INSUFFICIENCY
- Hydrocortisone bolus dosing 100 mg IV q8h
- Dexamethasone 8 mg IV daily

PERICARDIAL EFFUSION
- Will usually resolve without intervention when myxedema resolved

THYROID STORM

CLINICAL TIPS AND TRICKS

THYROID STORM
- Medical emergency
- Requires ICU admission
- Rare disorders
- Caused by inadequately controlled hyperthyroidism
- High risk of death

Causes
- Trauma
- Stress
- Infection
- Thyroid surgery
- Pregnancy

Assessment Findings

General
- Fever
  - Fever can be extreme, as high at 105
- Flushing
- Diaphoresis
- Exophthalmos
- Eyelid lag
- Infrequent blinking

Neurological
- Psychosis
- Stupor
- Delirium

Hemodynamics
- Tachycardia
- Atrial fibrillation
- Palpitation

Gastrointestinal
- Diarrhea
- Increase appetite
- Weight loss

Musculoskeletal
- Hyperreflexia

Diagnostics

Laboratory
- TSH
- T3 and T4
- Erythrocyte sedimentation rate (ESR)
- Antinuclear antibody (ANA)
- Chemistry
  - Hypercalcemia
- CBC
  - Anemia

Treatment and Management

Medications
- Propylthiouracil
- Methimazole

Hemodynamic Support
- Propranolol q4h

Fever Management
- Acetaminophen

CLINICAL TIPS AND TRICKS

EUTHYROID SICKNESS AND THYROID DYSFUNCTION OF THE CRITICALLY ILL

- Seen in critically ill patients
- May have low TSH and low T3 and T4
- Cytokines and inflammation can decrease TSH levels
- As patients recover from their critical illness, they may have a rise in TSH
- Euthyroid-sick patients will have an elevated reverse T3 and T4 showing adequate available hormone
- If reverse T3 and T4 are low, supplementation may be indicated

Bibliography

Ashton, N. (2005). Pituitary, adrenal and thyroid dysfunction. *Anesthesia Intensive Care Medicine, 6*(12), 346–349. https://doi.org/10.1383/anes.2005.6.10.346

Fliers, E., Bianco, A. C., Langouche, L., & Boelen, A. (2015). Thyroid function in critically ill patients. *Lancet Diabetes Endocrinol, 3*, 816. https://doi.org/10.1016/S2213-8587(15)00225-9

Holcome, S. S. (2005). Detecting thyroid disease. *Nursing, 35*(10), 4–9.

Jonklaas, J., Bianco, A. C., Bauer, A. J., Burman, K. D., Cappola, A. R., Celi, F. S., Cooper, D. S., Kim, B. W., Peeters, R. P., Rosenthal, M. S., & Sawka, A. M. (2014). Guidelines for the treatment of hypothyroidism: Prepared by the American thyroid association task force on thyroid hormone replacement. *Thyroid, 24*(12), 1670. https://doi.org/10.1089/thy.2014.0028

McCance, K. L., & Huether, S. E. (2019). *Pathophysiology: The biologic basis for disease in adults children* (8th ed.). Mosby.

Willis, G., Alhisabs, S., & Glouser, J. (2017). The great mimicker: Thyroid emergencies. *Investigative Medial Alert, 20*(9), 5–18.

SECTION VII

MANAGEMENT OF INFECTIOUS DISEASES

17

SEPSIS AND SEPTIC SHOCK

Causes

Infection
- Bacteria
- Fungus
- Yeast
- Viruses

Patients at Increased Risk for Sepsis
- Diabetes
- HIV/AIDS
- Chronic obstructive pulmonary disease (COPD)
- Cancer
- Chemotherapy
- Immunosuppressive drugs
- Solid organ transplant
- Extremes of age

Common Source of Infection
- Pneumonia
- Most common source of infection
- Intraabdominal Infection
- Infections of the urinary tract
- Wounds
- Invasive lines
- Meningitis

Assessment Findings

General
■ Fever
■ Ill appearance
■ Cold clammy skin
■ Hot dry skin
■ Reports symptoms consistent with active infection

Cardiovascular
■ Tachycardia
■ Hypotension
  ● Systolic blood pressure (SBP) <90
  ● Mean arterial pressure (MAP) <70
■ Elevated cardiac index (CI)
■ Low central venous pressure (CVP)

Pulmonary
■ Shortness of breath
■ Tachypnea
■ Respiratory failure
■ Cough
  ● Especially when pneumonia is the source

Renal
■ Decreased urine output
■ Acute oliguria
  ● Urine output less than 0.5 mL/kg/hr

Genitourinary
■ Dysuria
■ Frequency
■ Cloudy urine
■ Foul-smelling urine

Gastrointestinal
■ Hypoactive or absent bowel sounds
■ Nausea
■ Vomiting

Neuro
■ Altered mental status
■ Obtunded
■ Confusion
  ● May be early symptom in older adults

Integumentary
■ Cellulitis
■ Open wounds
■ Pressure wounds
■ Rash
■ Punctures

Endocrine
- Reports of hyperglycemia

CLINICAL TIPS AND TRICKS

SEVERITY SCREENING FOR SEPSIS
- Systemic inflammatory response syndrome (SIRS) criteria
  - Respiratory rate
  - White blood cell (WBC)
  - Bands
  - Temperature
  - Heart rate
  - $PaCO_2$
- Sequential Organ Failure Assessment Score
  - P/F ratio
  - Glasgow Coma Scale
  - MAP
  - Creatinine
  - Bili
  - Platelets
- Logistic Organ Dysfunction Score
  - P/F ratio
  - Glasgow Coma cale
  - MAP
  - Bili
  - Platelets
  - Urine output
  - Prothrombin time (PT)
  - Creatinine
- qSOFA
  - Respiratory rate
  - Glasgow Coma Scale
  - Systolic blood pressure

Diagnostics

Laboratory Findings
- CBC
  - WBCs >12 or <4
  - Bandemia >10%
  - Decrease platelets
- Chemistry
  - Elevated glucose without history of diabetes
  - Elevated BUN and creatinine
    - Creatinine increased >0.5 than baseline
- Lactate >2 mmol/L

- Coagulation
  - Elevated PT
  - Elevated PTT
  - Decreased fibrinogen
- Elevated procalcitonin level
  - Data support use in de-escalation of antibiotics and not as confirmation of sepsis
- Elevated CRP (C-reactive protein)
- Urinalysis
  - If source consistent with infection
    - Color: Dark
    - Clarity: Hazy
    - Bacteria/yeast: 1 to 4+
    - Nitrites: Positive
    - WBC: Present
    - Leukocyte esterase: Present
- Arterial blood gas (ABG)
  - P/F ratio <300
  - Metabolic acidosis
- Mixed venous blood gas
  - SpO_2 >70%

Radiology
- Chest x-ray
  - Pneumonia
  - Adult respiratory distress syndrome (ARDS)

CLINICAL TIPS AND TRICKS

COMMON BACTERIA SEEN IN SEPSIS
- Gram-positive bacteria
  - Staphylococcus aureus
  - Streptococcus pneumoniae
- Gram negative
  - Escherichia coli
  - Klebsiella species
  - Pseudomonas aeruginosa

Treatment and Management

Initial Treatment in Suspected Sepsis (first 3 hours)
- Fluid resuscitation for hypotension
  - Crystalloid bolus of 30 mL/kg
    - Actual body weight should be used
  - Hetastarch formulas should be avoided
- Obtain blood cultures
  - Ideally before antibiotics

■ Broad-spectrum antibiotics
  ● Ideally in the first 1 hour of identification of sepsis
  ● Make sure suspected sources are covered by therapy being initiated
    ■ Commonly vancomycin **and**
    ■ Piperacillin/tazobactam OR cefepime OR a carbapenem
■ Supplemental oxygen
  ● Sepsis often causes increased oxygen demand
  ● Titrate for optimal SpO_2 or PaO_2
  ● Intubation for respiratory distress

Management of Body Systems During Sepsis
■ Fever
  ● Acetaminophen
  ● Nonsteroidal anti-inflammatory drugs (NSAIDs)
  ● Cooling measures
    ■ Cooling pad
    ■ Cooling catheters
    ■ Cool fluids
■ Infectious disease
  ● Broad-spectrum antibiotics
  ● Evaluate risk for Methicillin-resistant *Staphylococcus aureus*
    ■ Chronically ill
    ■ Nursing home resident
    ■ Prisoner or recent incarceration
  ● Evaluate for atypical infections
    ■ Organ transplant
    ■ HIV/AIDS
  ● Evaluate for risk of fungal infections
  ● Immunocompromised patients
  ● Receiving chemo therapy
  ● Large cutaneous burns
■ Cardiovascular and shock
  ● Fluid resuscitation
    ■ Crystalloid bolus of 30 mL/kg
    ■ Continue if patient continues to respond hemodynamically
    ■ If large volumes required, may consider switching to albumin
    ■ Goal of CVP >12 but higher if intubated
    ■ Follow for increase in urine output
    ■ Follow for decrease in serum lactate
  ● Vasopressors
    ■ Use when patient is no longer responsive to fluid bolus or critically hypotensive
      ● Goal mean arterial pressure between 65 and 70 mmHg
    ■ Norepinephrine is recommended as first agent
    ■ Vasopressin can be added if patient requiring high doses of norepinephrine

- Dopamine should be avoided unless significant bradycardia, which is unusual
- Angiotensin II (Giapreza)
  - May be considered in nonresponsive hypotension after other pressor failure
  - May not be available in all centers
- Arterial catheter should be considered in all patients requiring vasopressor titration

CLINICAL TIPS AND TRICKS

NEW KID ON THE BLOCK: ANGIOTENSIN II

- New vasopressor
- Synthetic angiotensin II sold under trade name Giapreza
- Used for refractory shock in sepsis
- Increases systemic blood pressure due to vasoconstriction
- Indicated in hypotension not responsive to other pressors
- Common side effects include atrial fibrillation and other arrhythmias

- Pulmonary
  - Risk for respiratory failure
  - Follow ABG for hypoxemia
  - High risk of requiring intubation
  - Low tidal volume strategies recommended due to increased risk of ARDS
- Renal
  - Acute kidney injury is seen in more than 50% of patients with sepsis and is linked to an increase in mortality
  - Follow serial chemistries for renal function
  - Follow urine output
  - Patient may require renal replacement therapy due to renal injury
- Gastrointestinal (GI)
  - Ileus
  - Nasogastric or orogastric tube to low intermittent wall suction
  - If GI tract nonfunctioning, consider IV route for medications
  - Liver dysfunction
- Hematology
  - Coagulopathy
    - Fresh frozen plasma
    - Vitamin K
    - Cryoprecipitate
  - Anemia
    - Transfuse packed red blood cells
    - Usually to keep hgb >7

- ■ Neuro
  - ● Encephalopathy
  - ● Follow acidosis and liver dysfunction for possible causes of acute encephalopathy
- ■ Adrenal
  - ● Adrenal insufficiency in septic shock
  - ● Hydrocortisone replacement
    - ■ Generally, IV dosed q8 to 12h
    - ■ Seen as a late complication of sepsis and the critically ill

Bibliography

Angus, D. C., & van der Poll, T. (2013). Severe sepsis and septic shock. *Critical Care Medicine, 369*(9), 840–851. https://doi.org/10.1056/NEJMra1208623

Dellinger, R. P., Levy, M. M., Rhodes, A., Annane, D., Gerlach, H., Opal, S. M., Sevransky, J. E., Sprung, C. L., Douglas, I. S., Jaeschke, R., Osborn, T. M., Nunnally, M. E., Townsend, S. R., Reinhart, K., Kleinpell, R. M., Angus, D. C., Deutschman, C. S., Machado, F. R., Rubenfeld, G. D., … Moreno, R.; Surviving Sepsis Campaign Guidelines Committee including the Pediatric Subgroup (2013). Surviving sepsis campaign: International guidelines for management of severe sepsis and septic shock: 2013. *Intensive Care Medicine, 41*, 580–637. https://doi.org/10.1097/CCM.0b013e31827e83af

Gaileski, D. F., Mikkelsen, M. E., Band, R. A., Pines, J. M., Massone, R., Furia, F. F., Shofer, F. S., & Goyal, M. (2010). Impact of time to antibiotics on survival in patients with severe sepsis or septic shock in whom early goal-directed therapy was initiated in the emergency department. *Critical Care Medicine, 38*(4), 1045–1053. https://doi.org/10.1097/CCM.0b013e3181cc4824

Gupta, S., Sakhuja, A., Kumar, G., McGrath, E., Nanchal, R. S., & Kashani, K. B. (2016). Culture-negative severe sepsis. *Chest, 150*(6), 1251–1259. https://doi.org/10.1016/j.chest.2016.08.1460

Hohn, A., Balfer, N., Heising, B., Hertel, S., Wiemer, J. C., Hochreiter, M., & Schröder, S. (2018). Adherence to a procalcitonin-guided antibiotic treatment protocol in patients with severe sepsis and septic shock. *Annals of Intensive Care, 68*(8), 1–10. https://doi.org/10.1186/s13613-018-0415-5

Howell, M. D., & Davis, A. M. (2017). Management of sepsis and septic shock. *JAMA, 317*(8), 847–848. https://doi.org/10.1001/jama.2017.0131

Kaukonen, K., Bailey, M., Suzuki, S., Pilcher, D., & Bellomo, R. (2014). Mortality related to severe sepsis and septic shock among critically ill patients in Australia and New Zealand, 2000–2012. *JAMA, 311*(13), 1308–1316. https://doi.org/10.1001/jama.2014.2637

Kaukonen, K., Bailey, M., Suzuki, S., Pilcher, D., Cooper, J. D., & Bellomo, R. (2015). Systemic inflammatory response syndrome criteria in defining severe sepsis. *New England Journal of Medicine, 372*(17), 1629–1638. https://doi.org/10.1056/NEJMoa1415236

Marik, P. E., Khangoora, V., Rivera, R., Hooper, M. H., & Catravas, J. (2016). Hydrocortisone, vitamin C, and thiamine for the treatment of severe sepsis and septic shock. *Chest, 151*(6), 1229–1236. https://doi.org/10.1016/j.chest.2016.11.036

Puskarich, M. A., Marchick, M. R., Kline, J. A., Steuerwald, M. T., & Jones, A. E. (2009). One year mortality of patients treated with an emergency department based early goal directed therapy protocol for severe sepsis and septic shock: A before and after study. *Critical Care, 13*(5), R167. https://doi.org/10.1186/cc8138

Raith, E. P., Udy, A. A., Bailey, M., McGloughlin, S., MacIsaac, C., Bellomo, R., & Pilcher, D. V.; Australian and New Zealand Intensive Care Society (ANZICS) Centre for Outcomes and Resource Evaluation (CORE). (2017). Prognostic accuracy of the SOFA score, SIRS criteria, and qSOFA score for in-hospital mortality amount adults with suspected infection admitted to the intensive care unit. *JAMA, 317*(3), 290–300. https://doi.org/10.1001/jama.2016.20328

Seymour, C. W., Liu, V. X., Iwashyna, T. J., Brunkhorst, F. M., Rea, T. D., Scherag, A., Rubenfeld, G., Kahn, J. M., Shankar-Hari, M., Singer, M., Deutschman, C. S., Escobar, G. J., & Angus, D. C. (2016). Assessment of clinical criteria for sepsis: For the third international consensus definitions for sepsis and septic shock (Sepsis-3). *JAMA, 315*(8), 762–774. https://doi.org/10.1001/jama.2016.0288

18

FEVER OF UNKNOWN ORIGIN AND NOSOCOMIAL INFECTIONS

Causes

- Infection
  - Bacterial
    - Intraabdominal abscess
    - Appendicitis
    - Cholecystitis
    - Diverticulitis
    - Endocarditis
    - Pelvic inflammatory disease
    - Liver abscess
    - Osteomyelitis
    - Sinusitis
  - Specific bacteria
    - Lyme disease
    - Chlamydia
    - Mycoplasma
    - Syphilis
    - Tick-borne illnesses
    - Tuberculosis
  - Fungal
    - Aspergillosis
    - Candidiasis
    - Cryptococcosis
    - Histoplasmosis
  - Viral
    - Coxsackievirus
    - Cytomegalovirus (CMV)
    - Epstein–Barr virus (EBV)
    - Hepatitis (A, B, C, D, E)
    - Herpes simplex (HSV)
    - HIV
  - Parasitic
    - Giardia

- Neoplasm
  - Malignant lymphoma (most common)
  - Leukemia
- Vasculitis syndromes
- Granulomatous disorders
- Autoimmune disorders
  - Rheumatoid arthritis
  - Lupus
- Drug-induced fever
  - Drug reaction with eosinophilia and systemic symptoms (DRESS)

CLINICAL TIPS AND TRICKS

DRESS

- Rare but potentially fatal drug reaction
- Delayed onset of reaction
- Delay can be between 2 and 10 weeks from last dose of offending agent
- Clinical manifestations include cutaneous rash, atypical lymphocytes, and lymphadenopathy

Assessment Findings

CLINICAL TIPS AND TRICKS

FEVER: HISTORY-TAKING TIPS

- History and review of systems is key to identifying underlying cause:
  - History of recent travel
  - Animal contacts
    - Exotic pets
    - Job that requires animal work
    - Wild-animal encounters
  - Immunosuppression
  - Home medications
  - Detailed review of systems
    - Explore all positives for clarity
  - Follow patterns of organ involvement

- **Fever (101 F)**
- **Illness lasting greater than 2 to 3 weeks**
- **Tachycardia**
- **Ill appearing**
- **Hypotension**
- **Complaints specific to etiology**

CLINICAL TIPS AND TRICKS

FACTIOUS FEVER
- Fever falsely elevated by the patient
- Suspected when no suspected source or no other hemodynamic changes
- Seen more in females with healthcare knowledge
- May be symptom of Munchausen syndrome

Diagnostics

CLINICAL TIPS AND TRICKS

INITIAL WORKUP OF FEVER
- Complete blood count (CBC) with differential
- Serum chemistries
- Liver functions
- Lactic
- Chest x-ray
- Blood cultures

Laboratory
- CBC
  - Ideally with manual differential
- Chemistries
- Lactic
- Lactate dehydrogenase
- Interferon gold
  - If tuberculosis is suspected
- Inflammatory markers
  - C-reactive protein (CRP)
  - Eosinophil (ESR or sedimentation rate)
  - Antinuclear antibodies (ANA)
  - Rheumatoid factor
- Hepatitis panel (A, B, C)
  - Indicated when there are abnormal liver functions, or
  - Suspected exposure
- HIV
  - Indications
  - Risk factors present
  - Low cd4/cd8 count
  - Other opportunist infections

Blood cultures
- Ideally obtained from two different locations
- If possible, obtain when fever present
- Obtain set prior to initiation of antibiotics

Wound cultures
- If wounds present

Urinalysis and urine culture
Radiology
- Chest x-ray
- Right upper quadrant ultrasound
  - Evaluate liver and gallbladder
  - If liver functions abnormal
- CT abdomen and pelvis
  - If abdominal abscess or intrabdominal process suspected

ECHOCARDIOGRAM
- Suspected or concerns of endocarditis

Lumbar puncture
- Indicated when symptoms of central nervous system (CNS) infection, or
- If no other source is found

Punch biopsy
- May be indicated if a rash is present

Bone marrow biopsy
- Suspected malignancy

Treatment and Management

Ultimate treatment will be determined based on identification of underlying disease or disorder.

- **Fever management**
  - Follow fever curve and peak times
  - Follow fever in relationship to symptoms
  - Fever control for high fever
    - Medications
      - Acetaminophen
      - Nonsteroidal antiinflammatory drugs (NSAIDs)
    - Nonpharmacological
      - Cooling pad/blanked
      - Cooling catheter
      - Cooling esophageal tube
      - Cool intravenous (IV) fluids
- **Consider consultants**
  - Hematology and oncology

- Infectious disease
- Other specialties as indicated

NOSOCOMIAL INFECTIONS

CENTRAL LINE BLOODSTREAM INFECTION

Causes

- *Gram-positive bacteria*
  - *Staphylococcus*
    - Including methicillin-resistant *Staphylococcus aureus* (MRSA)
  - *Streptococcus*
  - *Enterococcus*
- *Gram-negative bacteria*
  - *Klebsiella*
  - *Enterobacter*
  - *Pseudomonas*
- *Fungal*
  - *Candida*

Assessment Findings

- Fever
- Chills
- Tachycardia
- Redness drainage at insertion site
- Extending cellulitis
- Hypoglycemia
  - Seen in systemic fungal infections
- Ill appearing
- Shock
- Sepsis

Diagnostics

Laboratory
- CBC
  - Leukocytosis
    - Trend from start of fever or suspected worsening of illness
  - Thrombocytopenia
- Chemistry
  - Rising creatinine
- Lactic
  - Elevated as sepsis marker

Blood cultures
- One from suspected line
- One from peripheral stick
- Ideally prior to initiation of antibiotics

Treatment and Management

- Remove central line if possible
- Central line holiday and peripheral access if appropriate for patient
- Broad-spectrum antibiotics
- Symptom management
  - Follow sepsis criteria
  - Fever management

CATHETER-ASSOCIATED URINARY TRACT INFECTION

Causes

- *Gram-negative bacteria*
  - *Escherichia coli*
  - *Klebsiella*
  - *Pseudomonas*
  - *Proteus*
- *Gram-positive bacteria*
  - *Staphylococcus epidermis*
  - *Staphylococcus aureus*
    - Including MRSA
  - *Enterococcus faecalis*
- *Yeast*
  - Less common

Risk Factors

- Advanced age
- Females
- Diabetes

Assessment Findings

- Pyuria
- Suprapubic discomfort
- Dysuria
- Sudden fever
- Flank pain
- Signs of sepsis without source

CLINICAL TIPS AND TRICKS

BACTERIURIA VERSUS INFECTION

Bacteriuria: Bacteria present in the urine. Presence of bacteria alone does not indicate infection. Bacteria presence without symptom of infection generally does not require treatment. Commonly seen from specimen contamination and in patients with colonization.

ASYMPTOMATIC BACTERIURIA SHOULD BE TREATED IN THE FOLLOWING POPULATIONS:

- Pregnant patients
- Patients undergoing renal transplant
- Patients undergoing urological procedures

Diagnostics

Laboratory
- CBC
  - Leukocytosis
    - Trend from start of fever or suspected worsening of illness
- Urinalysis and culture
  - Culture generally not treated unless >100,000 colonies or other indications that urinary tract is the source of infection

Treatment and Management

CLINICAL TIPS AND TRICKS

INDICATIONS FOR FOLEY CATHETER IN THE INPATIENT

- Acute and chronic urinary retention
- Accurate I&O during critical illness
- Bladder irrigation
- Traumatic injuries that limit mobility
  - Multiple fractures
  - Unstable pelvic fracture
- Perioperative phase for urological or gynecological procedures
- To promote wound healing to sacrum or perineum
- Comfort during end of life

Determine extent of infection
- Cystitis
  - No systemic symptoms
- Complicated urinary tract infection (UTI)
  - Systemic symptoms

- Chills
- Rigors
- Malaise
- The elderly may be more difficult to assess
  - May have increased confusion
  - Increased risk for falls
  - However, symptoms may indicate other pathology
- Signs of upper tract infection
  - Flank pain
  - Nausea and vomiting
  - Costovertebral tenderness
- Treatment
  - Evaluate risk of resistance
  - No risk of resistance
    - Ceftriaxone 1 g daily or piperacillin–tazobactam 3.375 g q6h
  - Risk of resistance
    - Gram-negative resistance
      - Carbapenem
        - Meropenem 1 g q8h
        - Doripenem 500 mg q8h
    - Gram-positive resistance
      - Vancomycin
        - Dosing based on weight and renal function
      - Daptomycin 4 to 6 mg/kg IV
      - Linezolid 600 mg IV q12h

CLINICAL TIPS AND TRICKS

RISK FACTORS FOR BACTERIAL RESISTANCE

- Previous resistant bacteria UTI
- Recent broad-spectrum antibiotic therapy
- Long-term antibiotic therapy
- Frequent UTIs
- Recent urological procedure

Other Assessments
- Assess need for catheter
- Discontinue foley if appropriate
- Change foley if unable to be discontinued
- Evaluate risk factors for resistant infection

Ventilator-Associated Pneumonia

Causes

- Pneumonia that occurs more than 48 hours after the initiation of mechanical ventilation
- Gram-positive bacteria
  - *S. aureus*
- Gram-negative bacteria
  - *Pseudomonas aeruginosa*
  - Other gram-negative bacilli

Assessment Findings

- Fever
- Tachypnea
- Increased secretions
- Purulent secretions
- Increased inspiratory pressures on ventilator
- Decreased tidal volumes
- Hypoxia
- Increased oxygen demand
- Bronchospasm

Diagnostics

Laboratory
- CBC
  - Increased leukocytosis

Radiology
- Chest x-ray
  - New or worsening infiltrate

Bronchoscopy
- Bronchoalveolar lavage
  - Allows for sampling of lower airways for culture

Treatment and Management

- Best treatment is prevention
  - Many places use ventilator-associated pneumonia (VAP) bundles to decrease risks of infection.
- Antibiotic therapy
  - Piperacillin–tazobactam or
  - Cefepime or
  - Levofloxacin or
  - Plus, vancomycin or linezolid if MRSA is suspected
- Bronchodilators
  - Albuterol or albuterol atrovent combination q4 to 6h
- Manage hypoxemia
  - Increase in FiO_2
  - Increase PEEP
- Fever management

CLINICAL TIPS AND TRICKS

VAP PREVENTION BUNDLES

- Head of bed >30 degrees unless contraindicated
- Oral care q4h with chlorhexidine gluconate–based solution
- Decrease any breaks in ventilator circuit unless necessary
- Epiglottic suctioning if available
- Stress ulcer prophylaxis
- Deep vein thrombosis prophylaxis

RESISTANT BACTERIA TABLE			
BACTERIA	**COMMON SITES OF INFECTION**	**RISK FACTORS**	**TREATMENT**
MRSA	Skin abscesses Urinary tract Respiratory tract wounds Blood Endocarditis	Chronic illness IV drug use Antibiotic therapy Long-term care facility resident	Vancomycin Daptomycin (not for lung coverage) Linezolid Ceftaroline fosamil Doxycycline (for community-acquired MRSA) Clindamycin (for community-acquired MRSA)

Clostridium difficile	Lower GI tract	Antibiotic therapy	Orally dosed Vancomycin Flagyl Fecal transplant
VRE	Blood Urinary tact Endocarditis Meningitis	Chronic illness Hospitalization Long-term care facility resident Antibiotic therapy	Linezolid daptomycin Tigecycline Telavancin Multi-drug–resistant strains may require combination therapy
CRE	Respiratory tract Urinary tract	Advanced age Resident of long-term care facility Hospitalization Exposure to broad-spectrum antibiotics Immunosuppression Recent endoscopic procedure	Treated with combination therapy Aminoglycosides • Tobramycin • Amikacin Polymyxin Tigecycline Fosfomycin

CRE, carbapenem-resistant enterobacteriaceae; GI, gastrointestinal; IV, intravenous; MRSA, methicillin-resistant *Staphylococcus aureus*; VRE, vancomycin-resistant enterococcus.

Bibliography

Cunha, B.A., Lortholary, O., & Cunha, C. B. (2019). Fever of unknown origin: A clinical approach. *American Journal of Medicine, 128*(10), e1–e15. https://doi.org/10.1016/j.amjmed.2015.06.001

Davis, C. (2019). Catheter-associated urinary tract infection: Signs, diagnosis, prevention. *British Journal of Nursing, 28*(2), 96–100. https://doi.org/10.12968/bjon.2019.28.2.96

Horowitz, H. (2013). Fever of unknown origin or fever of too many origins? *New England Journal of Medicine, 368*(3), 197–199. https://doi.org/10.1056/NEJMp1212725

Ibn Saied W., Mourvillier, B., Cohen, Y., Ruckly, S., Reignier, J., Marcotte, G., Siami, S., Bouadma, L., Darmon, M., de Montmollin, E., Argaud, L., Kallel, H., Garrouste-Orgeas, M., Soufir, L., Schwebel, C., Souweine, B., Glodgran-Toledano, D., Papazian, L., & Timsit, J.-F.; OUTCOMEREA Study Group. (2019). A comparison of the mortality risk associated with ventilator-acquired bacterial pneumonia and non-ventilator ICU-acquired bacterial pneumonia. *Critical Care Medicine, 47*(3), 345. https://doi.org/10.1097/CCM.0000000000003553

Leuck, A. M., Wright, D., Ellingson, L., Kraemer, L., Kuskowski, M. A., & Johnson, J. R. (2012). Complications of Foley catheters: Is infection the greatest risk? *Journal of Urology, 187*(5), 1662–1666. https://doi.org/10.1016/j.juro.2011.12.113

Lo, E., Nicolle, L. E., Coffin, S. E., Gould, C., Maragakis, L. L., Meddings, J., Pegues, D. A., Pettis, A. M., Saint, S., & Yokoe, D. S. (2014). Strategies to prevent catheter-associated urinary tract infections in acute care hospitals: 2014 update. *Infect Control Hospital Epidemiology, 35*(5), 464–479. https://doi.org/10.1086/675718

McCance, K. L., & Huether, S. E. (2019). *Pathophysiology: The biologic basis for disease in adults children* (8th ed.). Mosby.

National Healthcare Safety Network. (2021, January). *Urinary tract infection (Catheter-Associated Urinary Tract Infection [CAUTI] and Non-Catheter-Associated Urinary TractInfection [UTI]) events.* http://www.cdc.gov/nhsn/PDFs/pscManual/7pscCAUTIcurrent.pdf

Nicolle, L. E. (2001). A practical guide to antimicrobial management of complicated urinary tract infection. *Drugs Aging, 18*(4), 243. https://doi.org/10.2165/00002512-200118040-00002

Parisi, M., Gerovasili, V., Dimopoulos, S., Kampisiouli, E., Goga, C., Perivolioti, E., Argyropoulou, A., Routsi, C., Tsiodras, S., & Nanas, S. (2016). Use of ventilator bundle and staff education to decrease ventilator associated pneumonia in intensive care patients. *Critical Care Nurse, 36*(5), e1–e7. https://doi.org/10.4037/ccn2016520

SECTION VIII

BILLING, ASSESSMENTS, AND DOCUMENTATION

Nichole Miller and Tish Myers

19

NOTE TEMPLATES

HISTORY AND PHYSICAL

Chief Complaint (CC)

- One word or very short phrase

History of Present Illness

- What has happened leading up to patient being evaluated
- Use OLD CARTS to guide information and interview

CLINICAL TIPS AND TRICKS

OLD CARTS

- ONSET
- LOCATION
- DURATION
- CHARACTER
- AGGRAVATING FACTORS
- RELIEVING FACTORS
- TIMING
- SEVERITY

- Subjective and objective information
- May include pertinent history

Medical History

- Any significant medical history

Surgical History

- Any surgical history

Allergies

- Drug
- Food
- Latex
- Include reaction to each medication/food if allergies are present

Home Medications

- Medication
- Dose
- Schedule

Social History

- Tobacco
- Alcohol
- Drug use
- Vaccine status
- Occupation

Family History

- Mother
- Father
- Siblings
- Grandparents

Review of Systems

General

- Fever
- Chills
- Weight loss
- Fatigue

Skin

- Rashes
- Lesions
- Changes in hair

Head/Neck

- Headache
- Dizziness
- Trauma

Eyes

- Vision changes
- Eye pain
- Photophobia

Ears

- Pain
- Drainage
- Vertigo

Nose
- Epistaxis
- Discharge
- Sneezing

Mouth/Throat
- Pain
- Exudate
- Oral ulcers

Cardiovascular
- Chest pain
- Palpitations
- Edema

CLINICAL TIPS AND TRICKS

INTERVIEW TECHNIQUES
- Open-ended questions will elicit more information than closed-ended questions.
- Avoid "why" questions. This can make patients defensive.
- Use active-listening skills.
- Avoid leading questions.

Pulmonary
- Dyspnea on exertion
- Cough
- Sputum
- Orthopnea

Breasts
- Drainage
- Pain

Gastrointestinal
- Nausea vomiting
- Hematemesis
- Abdominal pain
- Diarrhea
- Constipation
- Melena
- Change in bowel habits

Genitourinary
- Dysuria
- Frequency
- Hematuria
- Penile/vaginal discharge

Endocrine
- Temperature intolerance
- Polyuria
- Polydipsia
- Polyphagia

Musculoskeletal
- Arthralgias
- Myalgias
- Erythema/tenderness

Neurology
- Syncope
- Vertigo
- Weakness
- Numbness

Psychiatric
- Anxiety
- Mania
- Depression
- Suicide ideology

CLINICAL TIPS AND TRICKS

REVIEW OF SYSTEMS
- Information is subjective
- Is what the patient states
- May differ at times from physical assessment

Vital Signs
- Temperature
- Blood pressure
- Heart rate
- Respiratory rate
- SpO_2
- Central venous pressure (CVP)
- Cardiac index (CI)
- Cardiac output (CO)
- Systemic vascular resistance (SVR)

Laboratory and Diagnostic Data

- Include pertinent labs
- Include pertinent abnormal labs

Physical Exam

General
- Age
- Sex
- What does the patient look like?

Head, Eyes, Ears, Nose, and Throat
- Atraumatic normocephalic
- Mucus membrane assessment

Cardiovascular
- Rate rhythm
- Heart sounds
- Jugular vascular distention

Pulmonary
- Rate
- Rhythm
- Mechanical ventilation
  - Mode
  - Ventilator settings
- Lung auscultation
- Chest tubes

Gastrointestinal
- Abdomen
- Abdomen sign findings
  - Murphy
  - Cullen

Genitourinary
- Urine color
- Urine output
- Foley
- Vaginal/penile drainage
- Pelvic exam findings

Neurology
- Mental status
- Cranial nerves
- May not be able to assess fully in sedated/intubated patients

Musculoskeletal
- Extremity movement
- Edema
- Compartment pressure

Psychiatry
- Mental state

Diagnosis

■ Your diagnoses or differential

Plan

■ What are you going to do for each patient?

CLINICAL TIPS AND TRICKS

CONSULT NOTE

■ If working with a specialty service, you may be completing a consultation note instead of an H&P.

■ Consult notes are similar to H&P and contain all the same parts.

■ Physical exam may be more specific to the specialty (e.g., cardiology may have a focused assessment of the cardiovascular system).

■ Plan will also be more specific to the specialty and may not address all aspects of the patient's care.

OPERATIVE NOTE TEMPLATE

Start Date

Start Time

Pre-Procedure Diagnosis
● Why is the patient having this procedure done?

Post-Procedure Diagnosis
● What was found during the procedure?
● It can be the same as the preprocedural diagnosis or it could be different.

Procedure(s) Performed
● Name of surgical or other procedure performed

Primary Surgeon

Assistant(s)
● Should be identified by name and title

Anesthesia

Types
   ■ General
      ● Endotracheal
      ● Tracheostomy
   ■ LMA
   ■ Regional
   ■ Epidural or spinal
   ■ Local
   ■ Monitored anesthesia care (MAC)
   ■ Twilight or moderate sedation

Technique/Procedure
- Describe in detail the procedure performed.
- This section is often completed by the surgeon if the procedure is completed with a surgeon.

Specimens Removed
- Tissue sent to microbiology or pathology
- Body parts removed and disposition

Implants
- Name of or type of any implants such as orthopedic or plastics devices
- Include serial number of implanted products and lot number

Complications

Fluids
- Type of fluids given and amount infused
- Can include blood or blood products

Estimated Blood Loss
- Noted in milliliters

Findings
- Any important data about the procedure
- Often include measurements
- Tourniquet times
- Pump times
- Abnormal findings
- Exploration findings

DEATH SUMMARY TEMPLATE

Patient Identifiers
- Name
- Date of birth
- Medical record number

Date of Admission

Date of Death

Name of Attending Physician Notified

Name of Primary Care Physician
- Name of PCP if available
- Was the PCP notified of patient's death?

Names of Any Consulting Physicians
- Include here any other physicians who assisted in the patient's care while hospitalized other than the admitting physician

Date and Description of Operative or Other Procedures
- Include name of healthcare providers who completed the procedures if available

History of Present Illness
- Summarize why the patient was admitted to the hospital; include the following:

- Age and gender
  - Where patient was admitted from
  - ED
  - Direct admit
- Another facility
  - Reason for admission to include symptoms and any diagnoses if known

Course of Hospitalization

- Summarize pertinent laboratory and other diagnostic data
- Pertinent results of imaging such as computerized axial tomography (CAT) scans, MRIs, x-rays, and so forth
- Biopsy results
- Culture source and results
- What was the result or action performed in relation to these findings?
- Were antibiotics given? Were they completed?
- Unexpected or untoward occurrences and the outcome
- Description of events leading up to the patient's death
- Note if the patient expired within 24 hours of admission
- Note time of death
  - Note who pronounced the patient deceased

Diagnosis That Is Presumed to Be the Cause of Death

- Common examples
  - Cardiopulmonary arrest
  - Respiratory arrest
  - Shock

Name of Family Member Notified

- Was an autopsy requested by family?

Name of Medical Examiner Notified (If Applicable)

- Was an autopsy requested by the medical examiner?

Name of Funeral Home Notified

- Disposition of body (i.e., hospital morgue)

DISCHARGE SUMMARY

Name and Title of Person Dictating the Summary

- NPs and PAs state name of MD they are dictating on behalf of

Patient Identifiers

- Name
- Date of birth
- Medical record number

Date of Admission

- Specify date

Date of Discharge

- Specify date

Admitting Diagnosis
- Initial reason for admission to the hospital

Name of Attending Physician

Name of Primary Care Physician
- State "PCP unknown" if this is the case

Name of Referring Physician
- This is important information to include in the admission H&P and can be located there if available; otherwise, state "unknown."

Names of Any Consulting Physicians
- Include here any other physicians who assisted in the patient's care while hospitalized other than the admitting physician (also referred to as the "attending physician")

Date and Description of Operative or Other Procedures
- Include name of healthcare providers who completed the procedures if available

Brief History
- Summarize why the patient was admitted to the hospital and include the following:
- Age and gender
  - Where patient was admitted from
  - ED
  - Direct admit
- Outside facility
  - Reason for admission to include symptoms and any diagnoses if known

Hospital Course
- Summarize pertinent laboratory and other diagnostic data
- White blood cell (WBC) elevated
- Low hemoglobin
- Platelet counts (high or low)
- Abnormal chemistry results
- Results of CAT scans, MRIs, x-rays, and so forth
- Biopsy, urinalysis, or tissue culture results
- What was the result or action performed in relation to these findings
- Antibiotics
  - Unexpected or untoward occurrences and the outcome

Discharge Diagnosis or Diagnoses
- May be multiple depending on patient and length of stay

Patient Condition on Discharge
- Stable
- Improved
- Fair
- Guarded
- Critical

Discharge Medications
- Include name of drug, dosage, frequency, and duration of any new medications prescribed

- For narcotics, include quantity prescribed
- Include names of any usual home medications that may have been discontinued

Discharge Instructions
- Activity
- Weight-bearing status may be important for some patients
- Use of assistive devices
- Diet
- Restrictions or changes
- Other treatments such as wound care or care for surgical drains
- Dressings
- Foley catheter care
- Ostomy care
- Tracheostomy care
- Home health assistance ordered or ongoing
- Physical and occupational therapy (PT)/OT
- Aide
- Hospice
- Follow-up
- Name of provider
- Appointment date and time (if applicable)

SOAP PROGRESS NOTE

General

- Hospital day or postop day number
  - If postop, what was the procedure performed?

Subjective

- Chief complaint
  - Use patient's own words to describe how they feel
  - What do they report?
- Nursing reports
- Note any reported concerns, events, or changes in condition

Objective

- Vital signs
- I&O
- Weight or changes in weight
- Physical assessment data
  - General appearance
  - HEENT
  - Neck
  - Respiratory

- Cardiovascular
- Abdomen
- Genitourinary
- Musculoskeletal
- Neurological
- Psych
- Wounds/incisions
- Pertinent laboratory data
- Other diagnostic findings
- Treatment and prophylaxis
- Include pertinent changes to medications, antibiotics, lines or other invasive devices, ventilator, oxygen, tube feeds, intravenous fluids, and so forth

Diagnosis

- Any applicable diagnoses
- List and update all diagnosis

Assessment and Plan

- A descriptive plan of care to address each diagnosis
- Include discharge planning

20

BILLING FOR SERVICES

GENERAL INPATIENT ADMISSION CODES

99221—Detailed History of Physical

Time at bedside approximately 30 minutes

Presenting Problem Severity
- Low

Documentation Required
- Chief complaint
- History of present illness
- Review of systems
- Pertinent medical history
- Social history

Medical Decision-Making
- Not complex
- Minimal decision-making
- Very straightforward

CLINICAL TIPS AND TRICKS

BILLING
- Billing captures the services provided and allows reimbursement from insurance.
- These will vary by specialty, location, and supervision type.
- Location of patient does not mean they qualify for billing at that level.
- Some places validate positions by hours billed.
- Billing can be used to justify raises or bonuses.

99222—Comprehensive History and Physical

Time at bedside approximately 50 minutes

Presenting Problem Severity
- Moderate

Documentation Required
- Chief complaint
- History of present illness (HPI)
- Home medications

- Medical history
- Family medical history
- Social history
- Review of all body systems
- Physical exam

Medical Decision-Making
- Moderate
- Two of the following three must be met or exceeded:
  - Multiple number of diagnoses or management options
  - Moderate amount and/or complexity of data to be reviewed
  - Moderate risk of significant complications, morbidity, and/or mortality

99223—Comprehensive History and Physical

Bedside time approximately 70 minutes

Presenting Problem Severity
- High

Documentation Required
- Chief complaint
- HPI
- Home medications
- Medical history
- Family medical history
- Social history (tobacco, alcohol, drug use; vaccine status)
- Review of all body systems
- Physical exam

Medical Decision-Making
- High
- Two of the following three must be met or exceeded:
  - Extensive number of diagnoses or management options
  - Extensive amount and/or complexity of data to be reviewed
  - High risk of significant complications, morbidity, and/or mortality

SUBSEQUENT DAILY BILLING CODES

99231—Problem Focused

- Approximately 15 minutes at bedside
- Medical decision-making is low/straightforward

99232—Expanded Problem Focused

- Approximately 25 minutes
- Medical decision-making moderate

99233—Detailed

- Approximately 35 minutes
- Medical decision-making high or complex

OBSERVATION CODES

- Observation codes are used when a patient is not expected to spend greater than two nights in the hospital.
- Severity of patient condition can range from low to high in the same manner as a full inpatient admission.

99218—Detailed History and Exam for Observation Patient

Bedside time approximately 30 minutes

Presenting Problem Severity
- Low

Documentation Required
- Chief complaint
- HPI
- Home medications
- Medical history
- Family history
- Social history (tobacco, ETOH, drug use; vaccine status)
- Brief review of systems
- Physical exam

Medical Decision-Making
- Low or straightforward

99219—Comprehensive History and Exam for Observation Patient

Bedside time approximately 50 minutes of time

Presenting Problem Severity
- Moderate

Documentation Required
- Chief complaint
- HPI
- Medical history
- Family medical history
- Social history
- Review of all body systems

Medical Decision-Making
- Moderate
- Two of the following three must be met or exceeded:

- Multiple number of diagnoses or management options
- Moderate amount and/or complexity of data to be reviewed
- Moderate risk of significant complications, morbidity, and/or mortality

99220—Comprehensive History and Exam

Bedside time approximately 70 minutes

Presenting Problem Severity
- High

Documentation Required
- Chief complaint
- HPI
- Medical history
- Family medical history
- Social history (tobacco, ETOH, drug use; vaccine status)
- Review of all body systems

Medical Decision-Making
- High/complex
- Two of the following three must be met or exceeded:
  - Extensive number of diagnoses or management options
  - Extensive amount and/or complexity of data to be reviewed
  - High risk of significant complications, morbidity, and/or mortality

SUBSEQUENT DAILY BILLING CODES FOR OBSERVATION PATIENTS

- Codes used after hospital day 1
- Bill for daily care provided
- Patients requiring more than 3 days of daily billing should be changed to inpatient status for continued billing

Observation Subsequent Care

- **99224 Low**
- **99225 Moderate**
- **99226 High**

CLINICAL TIPS AND TRICKS

CONSULTING SERVICES
- Consults will be billed under a consult code 99251 to 99253.
- Initial consults should contain the same information as an H&P based on the acuity and complexity of the patient.
- Plan should reflect specialty.

CRITICAL CARE BILLING CODES

- Critical care time is billed by minutes.
- Initial H&P and daily care are billed under the same code.
- Billed at a minimum of 30 minutes.

99291 30 to 74 minutes

99292 Each additional 30 minutes (added to initial code)

- Both codes can be used together.

Documentation Required Every Hospital Day
- Chief complaint
- HPI
- Review of all body systems
- Physical exam
- Diagnosis to support need for ICU level of care
- Plan for each diagnosis

CLINICAL TIPS AND TRICKS

BILLABLE PROCEDURES
Many procedures are reimbursable.

- Central line placement
  - Peripherally inserted central catheter line
  - Central venous catheter
  - Dialysis catheter
- Arterial line placement
- Incision and drainage
- Laceration repair
- Chest tube placement
- Thoracentesis
- Paracentesis

INDEX

ventilator associated pneumonia,
  155–156
note templates
  consult note, 166
  death summary, 167–168
  discharge summary, 168–170
  history and physical, 161–166
  operative note, 166–167
  SOAP progress note, 170–171
NS. *See* normal saline
NSAIDs, 117, 143, 150
NSTEMI. *See* non-ST elevation
  myocardial infarction

observation codes, 175–176
obturator sign, 118
octreotide, for hepatorenal syndrome, 107
OLD CARTS, 161
operative note, 166–167
osmolality, calculated, 87

packed red blood cells (PRBC), transfusion of, 96, 100, 144
pamidronate, for hypercalcemia, 77
pantoprazole
  for esophageal varices, 98
  for peptic ulcer disease, 97
paracentesis, 105, 121
PCI. *See* percutaneous coronary intervention
pentobarbital, for intracranial hemorrhage, 47
peptic ulcer disease, 96–97
percutaneous coronary intervention
  (PCI), 8
pericardial effusion, 133, 134
peritoneal aspirate, 116
peritoneal dialysis, 119, 121
peritonitis, 119–121
permissive hypercapnia, 35
P/F ratio, 34
phosphorus
  hyperphosphatemia, 79–80
  hypophosphatemia, 80
  normal level, 79
  supplementation, 80
physical exam, 165
physiological shunt, 28
piperacillin, for sepsis, 143
piperacillin-tazobactam

for catheter associated urinary tract
  infection, 154
for ventilator associated pneumonia,
  156
polymyxin, for carbapenem resistant
  enterobacteriaceae, 157
portal hypertension, 105
postictal state, 51
postrenal acute kidney injury, 65–66
potassium
  hyperkalemia, 69–71
  hypokalemia, 71–72
  normal level, 69
  supplementation, for hypokalemia, 72
potassium chloride, for metabolic
  alkalosis, 88
prasugrel, for myocardial infarction, 7
PRBC. *See* packed red blood cells,
  transfusion of
prerenal acute kidney injury, 59–61
proliferative phase of adult respiratory
  distress syndrome, 33
prone positioning, for ARDS, 35–36
propofol, for intracranial hemorrhage, 47
propranolol, 135
  for esophageal varices, 98
propylthiouracil, for thyroid storm, 135
protamine sulfate, 47
proton pump inhibitors, for
  Mallory-Weiss tear, 98
pruritis, 105
psoas sign, 118
punch biopsy, 150

qSOFA score, 141

Ranson's criteria, 112
renal artery stenosis, 67–68
renal calculi, 65
renal failure, 59–66
renal replacement therapy, 61, 63
respiratory acidosis, 88–90
respiratory alkalosis, 90
respiratory failure, 27–31
  chest x-ray reading tips, 29–30
  intubation criteria, 31
review of systems (ROS), 162–164
rifaximin, for hepatic encephalopathy, 105
ROS. *See* review of systems
Rovsing's sign, 118

Printed in the United States
by Baker & Taylor Publisher Services